Advances in Cerebral Aneurysm Treatment

Edited by Alba Scerrati and Giorgio Mantovani

Published in London, United Kingdom

Advances in Cerebral Aneurysm Treatment
http://dx.doi.org/10.5772/intechopen.106102
Edited by Alba Scerrati and Giorgio Mantovani

Contributors
Sérgio Tadeu Fernandes, Edson Bernaldino Neto, Hugo Leonardo Doria-Netto, Revaz Dzhindzhikhadze, Andrey Polyakov, Renat Kambiev, Anton Ermolaev, Igor Bogdanovich, Andrey Zaitsev, Pasquale Anania, Pietro Fiaschi, Michelle P. Lin, Guilherme Nascimento de Morais, Salomón Rojas, Tsuyoshi Izumo, Luis Antonio Marín-Castañeda, Hector Eduardo Valdez-Ruvalcaba, Fernanda de Leon-Mendoza

First published in London, United Kingdom, 2023 by IntechOpen
IntechOpen is the global imprint of INTECHOPEN LIMITED, registered in England and Wales, registration number: 11086078, 5 Princes Gate Court, London, SW7 2QJ, United Kingdom

British Library Cataloguing-in-Publication Data
A catalogue record for this book is available from the British Library

Additional hard and PDF copies can be obtained from orders@intechopen.com

Advances in Cerebral Aneurysm Treatment
Edited by Alba Scerrati and Giorgio Mantovani
p. cm.
Print ISBN 978-1-83768-736-7
Online ISBN 978-1-83768-737-4
eBook (PDF) ISBN 978-1-83768-738-1

Meet the editors

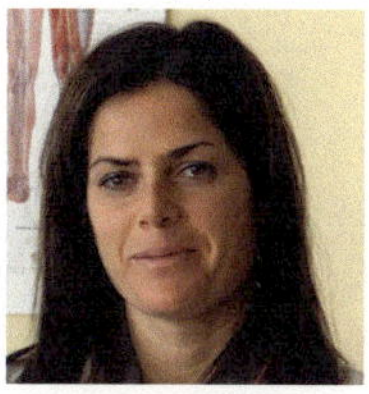

Dr. Alba Scerrati is an Assistant Professor of Neurosurgery, University of Ferrara, Italy, and a neurosurgeon at the University Hospital of Ferrara. She graduated from medical school in 2010 and completed her residency in neurosurgery at the Catholic University of Rome, Policlinico Gemelli. Her main scientific interests are skull base surgery and neurovascular surgery. She is working on the development of 3D printing techniques for neurovascular surgery training and simulation. She has participated in different clinical studies on cerebrovascular diseases and cerebrospinal fluid (CSF) dynamics. Dr. Scerrati is the author and co-author of more than eighty indexed publications.

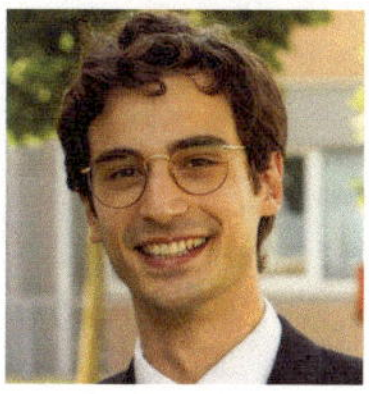

Dr. Giorgio Mantovani is a resident in the Neurosurgery Residency Program, University of Ferrara, Italy. He graduated from medical school in 2019. He has participated as a speaker and tutor at several international congresses and courses. He has led and participated in different clinical trials, mainly regarding cerebrovascular circulation, cerebrospinal fluid (CSF) dynamics, and functional neurosurgery for pain.

Contents

Preface

With the advancement of neuroimaging diagnostics and basic science research, numerous treatment options are now available in neurosurgery, and the choice of the most appropriate patient-tailored strategy becomes more difficult. This is especially true for cerebral aneurysms, a field of neurosurgery that experiences continuous and profound changes both in terms of approach and prognosis. For example, we are now dealing with an increasing number of patients who survive after an aneurysm' rupture and treatment, and with these patients comes the challenge of recurrent aneurysms and their implications. This book provides insight into new and emerging technologies and information that are pushing the boundaries and defining the landscape of cerebral aneurysm treatment.

Chapters 1–4 present some of the latest advancements, from the pathophysiology of early subarachnoid hemorrhage to the implementation of artificial intelligence into clinical practice. Chapters 5–7 discuss operative surgical management of a cerebral aneurysm, both on the first approach and during challenging recurrent surgery, highlighting the intraoperative tools that can help maximize patient safety.

This book is a valuable resource for experienced professionals as well as those approaching this topic for the first time.

Alba Scerrati and Giorgio Mantovani
Department of Neurosurgery,
University of Ferrara
Ferrara, Italy

Section 1

Basic Science

Chapter 1

A New Paradigm: How to Study the Exact Location of a Paraclinoid Aneurysm and the Cavernous Sinus in the Preoperative Stage through Imaging

Sérgio Tadeu Fernandes, Hugo Leonardo Dória-Netto and Edson Bernaldino Neto

Abstract

Intracranial aneurysms (IAs) found in the subarachnoid compartment of the internal carotid artery are at risk of rupturing and producing hemorrhage into this space, producing all the known serious pathological manifestations of subarachnoid hemorrhage. On the other hand, those who are exclusively in the intracavernous segment have this negligible risk. It is in this context that a peculiar class of IAs fits, the paraclinoid aneurysms, which are characterized by their complex anatomical relationships with the optic apparatus, anterior clinoid process, the first supraclinoidal arterial branches of the carotid artery, the oculomotor nerve and the segment mainly said clinoid, which is delimited by the proximal and distal dural rings. It is of crucial importance, and challenging, to determine the location of paraclinoid aneurysms and their exact relationship with the cavernous sinus, given the need to establish an adequate line of treatment for each case. Through preoperative studies of 3 t Magnetic Resonance, comparison with 3D bio models and microsurgical exploration, it was possible to accurately demarcate these anatomical relationships. Therefore, today it is possible to establish the accurate location of the paraclinoid aneurysm in relation to the cavernous sinus by means of MR images and to carry out an adequate, effective, and safe operative planning.

Keywords: paraclinoid, aneurysm, cavernous sinus, oculomotor, microsurgical anatomy

1. Introduction

Usually, arteries in the human body have 3 layers of tissue called, from the vascular lumen to the outermost layer, the intima, media, and adventitia, respectively. The intima is composed of an endothelial tissue layer, which has direct contact with intraluminal blood, and a subendothelial layer, formed by connective tissue. The internal elastic lamina, a layer of elastic fibers, separates the tunica intima from the tunica media. The media is basically formed by concentrically organized smooth muscle fibers and collagen fibers, in which type III collagen predominates. The external elastic lamina separates the tunica media and adventitia, typical in arteries throughout the body but absent in intracranial arteries. Finally, the adventitia is mainly formed by a complex network interspersed with type I collagen, elastin, fibroblasts, nerves, and vasa vasorum. Therefore, the wall of the cerebral arteries has a different structure from other extracranial arteries, with a scarce adventitia and a low proportion of elastic fibers. Furthermore, they are immersed in the cerebrospinal fluid of the subarachnoid space instead of the surrounding connective tissue [1, 2].

In normal arteries, myointimal hyperplasia is an adaptive physiological reaction to hemodynamic stress or to a mechanism of vascular injury, resulting from a change in the phenotype of smooth muscle cells in the tunica media, which promote their migration and proliferation, outlining the lesion endothelium [3]. Once the molecular mechanisms become unable to compensate for the myointimal injury, cellular and humoral inflammatory responses are triggered (mainly responsible for aneurysm formation) [4–6], and responses mediated by inflammatory cytokines, such as tumor necrosis factor (TNF).), interleukin-β (IL-1β) and matrix metalloproteinases (MMPs), which promote macrophage influx and continuous degradation of collagen and elastin fibers [6–9]. IA is, therefore, an encephalic vascular lesion characterized by an abnormal dilation of the blood vessels of the brain, affecting, in general, about 5% of the population [7, 10–13], resulting from a molecular and hemodynamic imbalance, the which would explain its formation in arterial junctions and bifurcations, where an excess of hemodynamic stress is exerted on the vessel wall, followed, then, by a local inflammatory process that leads to disruption of the internal elastic lamina [14–17].

Once the IA ruptures, blood leaks into the subarachnoid space, the natural space between the arachnoid mater and the pia mater, producing spontaneous subarachnoid hemorrhage (SAH). It is an entity with high mortality, reaching 50% of affected individuals, and considerable morbidity among survivors. It is noteworthy the fact that approximately 30% of subarachnoid hemorrhages resulting from intracranial aneurysm rupture occur during sleep. This denotes a multifactorial pathophysiological nature fundamentally related to inflammation and not exclusively hemodynamic, since in this period hemodynamic stress tends to be less intense than during the day. In the natural history of IA there are known modifiable and non-modifiable risk factors for rupture. As an example of the former, we can mention smoking and high blood pressure. Non-modifiable factors include advanced age, genetic profile, and family history of SAH, growth of the aneurysmal sac, among others [7, 13].

Bouthillier and van Loveren's classification (**Figure 1**), separates the internal carotid artery into segments according to its branches and anatomical relationships with adjacent structures. This makes it possible to classify carotid saccular ais according to these segments and their respective vessels. Thus, IA's can be in the cavernous, clinoid, ophthalmic and/or posterior communicating segments of the carotid artery and are primarily related to an arterial branch of the carotid artery or to an anatomical structure of interest.

As for the paraclinoid IAs, specifically, since 1968 with the work of Drake et al. [18], anatomical patterns are studied to try to classify them. However, until today we find confounding factors that add difficulty in understanding these classifications. Much of this stems from the fact that the existing nomenclature of aneurysms

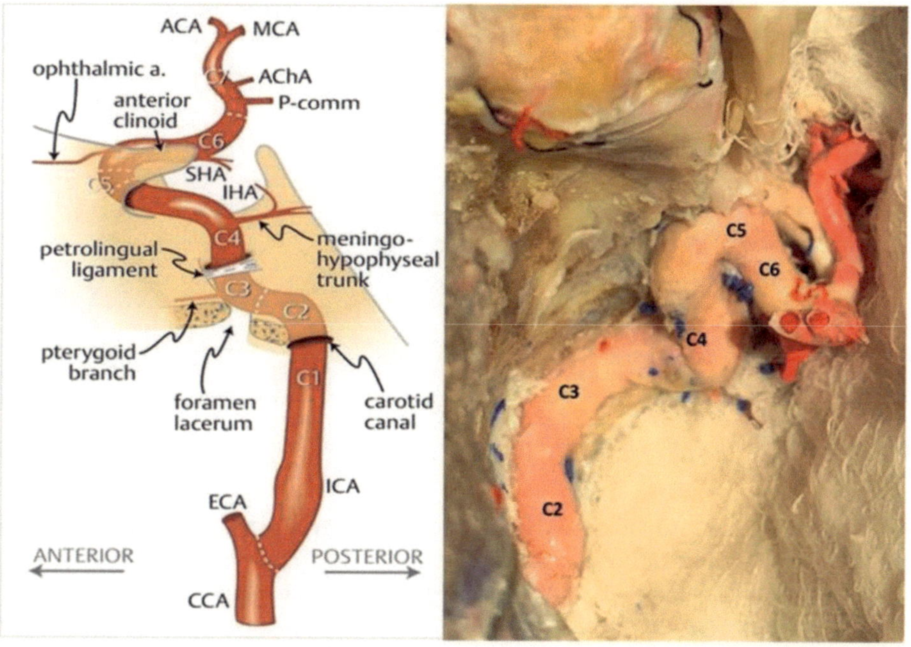

Figure 1.
Anatomical structure of the internal carotid artery (ICA). Segments: petrous (C2), lacerus (C3), cavernous (C4), clinoid (C5), ophthalmic (C6), proximal and distal dural rings, III cranial nerve and cavernous sinus. By the classification of Bouthhillier and van Loveren. On the left, schematic drawing and on the right, a piece obtained through anatomical dissection (adapted from Boutillier and Van Loveren left and right anatomical dissection by Hugo Doria, MD PhD).

arising from the clinoid and ophthalmic segments of the ICA is contradictory, mainly for anatomical reasons [19, 20]. First: the ophthalmic artery can arise both from the clinoid segment (C5) and from the ophthalmic segment (C6) [21] of the ICA as previously exposed [12, 19]. Second: aneurysms in this region do not necessarily arise in relation to a named arterial branch [19, 20]. Third: aneurysms in this area can be intradural, extradural or transitional and sometimes it is impossible to make this determination using radiographic investigations currently available [20]. Fourth: the recognition of the carotid cavum as an entity further complicated the issue, as cavum aneurysms are located below the plane of the distal dural ring (DDR), but are intradural [20, 22, 23]. In a summarized and practical way, the proposed classifications try to establish some standard for the surgical technique, always in search of the basic principles of the management of cerebral aneurysms, regardless of their location (establishing proximal and distal vascular control; adequate exposure of the neck and complete obliteration of the aneurysm with maintenance of cerebral blood flow distal to the aneurysm) [23].

Paraclinoid aneurysms are lesions that originate in the cavernous, clinoid, or ophthalmic segments of the ICA, defined by Bouthillier as segments C4, C5 and C6, respectively (**Figure 2**).

These are aneurysms that may arise proximally to the proximal dural ring (PDR), between the dural rings or distally to the DDR, between the distal dural ring and the posterior communicating artery and may be intra or extracavernous. Extracavernous paraclinoid aneurysms present a risk of SAH and usually require treatment, while unequivocally intracavernous aneurysms are located completely below the proximal

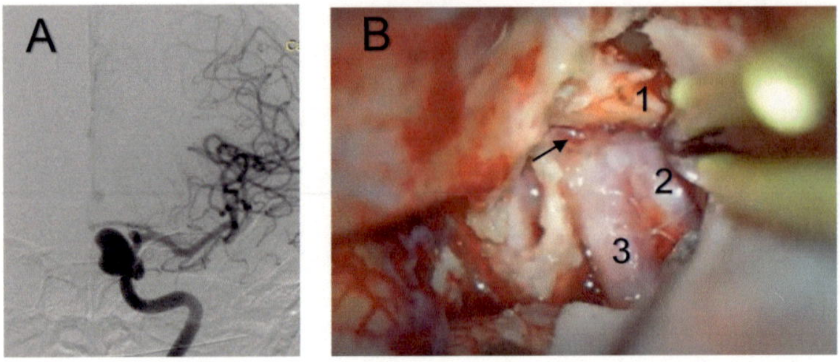

Figure 2.
A - Angiography with digital subtraction in the AP showing a large multi-lobulated paraclinoid aneurysm with a medial conformation. B – Microsurgical image of the same aneurysm after anterior intradural clinoidectomy. 1 – Optic Nerve, 2 – Aneurysm, 3 – Left Carotid Artery, black arrow – emergence of the ophthalmic artery (angiography and microsurgical photography kindly provided by Sergio Tadeu Fernandes, MD PhD).

dural ring, rarely coursing with SAH and present lower morbidity than aneurysms originating from the intradural space [24].

Approximately 33–59% of paraclinoid IAs are associated with the ophthalmic artery; 27–47% are associated with the superior hypophyseal artery and between 14% and 20% are not associated with any arterial branch. Paraclinoid IAs comprise between 1.4% to 9.1% of all ruptured aneurysms [25].

They are considered uncommon, accounting for approximately 5% of IAs, reaching up to 14% of IAs, in some studies, with an increased prevalence in women [26–28]. These aneurysms affect the ICA between the cavernous segment and the origin of the posterior communicating artery.

As for the diagnosis, the available methods are classified as invasive and non-invasive. The invasive method is digital subtraction angiography (DSA) performed in a hemodynamic suite through selective arterial catheterization of the intracranial vascular tree, which allows, in addition to the structural study, the analysis of hemodynamic behavior in real time. Despite being invasive and with intrinsic risks, this method is still consolidated as the gold standard for this purpose [29, 30]. On the other hand, non-invasive methods include the use of images processed by computer graphics and three-dimensional reconstructions obtained by Computed Tomography (CT-Angio) or Magnetic Resonance (MR-Angio) devices that are increasingly sensitive and specific, often used not only as screening, but replacing DSA in selected cases with the additional benefit of contributing, not only with the visualization of the target pathology, but its relationships with adjacent structures, such as the anterior clinoid process [31, 32].

However, despite all the technological advances and modern imaging techniques validated so far, both by invasive and non-invasive methods, paraclinoid aneurysms still represent a separate challenge. In view of the difficulty in determining whether the aneurysm studied is located exclusively in the cavernous compartment of the carotid artery, or whether it has a relationship, even if partial, with the subarachnoid space. The practical significance of such information is that each type of aneurysm requires a different surgical strategy. Aneurysms identified as being completely intradural may not require anterior clinoidectomy. On the other hand, transitional aneurysms may require a wide opening of the dural rings and adequate management of the roof of the cavernous sinus. Still, those located completely in the intracavernous space rarely require any kind of approach. Until then, it was only possible to determine this exact relationship through microsurgical exploration.

Many strategies have emerged with the purpose of resolving this dilemma. The proposal to use the origin of the ophthalmic artery as a marker for the intradural ICA, making a distinction between the intra and extradural segments, had some relevance, but it was soon found that this anatomical marker had low accuracy, since the origin of the artery Ophthalmic is extradural, that is, proximal to the distal dural ring, in 2–16% of cases [11, 12, 19, 23, 33–35]. There was a proposal to use the base of the ACP in lateral radiographs, serving as a more reliable marker than the origin of the OphA in angiograms, which also proved to be of low accuracy because, for example, carotid cavum aneurysms can be observed below the level of the ACP and, even so, they are inside the intradural space. Subsequently, Oikawa *et al.* [36] proposed that the use of the anterior clinoid process (ACP) in lateral projection radiographs should be replaced by the sellar tubercle in the same projection, when evaluating aneurysms on the medial side of the dural ring, as this is more proximal than the lateral one [36]. Kim *et al.* stated that they were not aware of any combination of radiographic exams that allowed the reliable identification of the distal dural ring, reaffirming that "surgical exploration is the only solution in these cases" [19]. In 2001, Murayama *et al.* proposed the use of 3D CTA as an indirect method for identifying the distal dural ring, noting that in 84.8% of the evaluated images it was possible to identify a concave impression on the anterior curve of the ICA and suggested that this concavity coincides with the location of the distal dural ring, because of ring fixation to the ICA [37]. Gonzalez *et al.* postulated that, if the optic pillar could be reliably identified with high-resolution CTA, it could represent an anatomical landmark for evaluating aneurysms in this critical region [24]. Hashimoto *et al.* applied the same methodology for analysis of the optical pillar, through CTA images, comparing images and intra-operative findings and stated that the optical pillar is the most useful landmark for operative planning of aneurysms in this region [38].

With the purpose of changing the indirect reference of the dural rings previously studied by previous methods, magnetic resonance imaging (MRI) begins to be used for direct visualization of the distal dural ring and the limits of the cavernous sinus in relation to paraclinoid aneurysms. However, the method initially ran into difficulties such as low spatial resolution and the need to improve signal acquisition powers. Thines *et al.* proposed the improvement of the resolution in 3 Tesla weighted in T2, demonstrating in thin and contiguous sections, the dural folds of the roof of the cavernous sinus and the distal dural ring, however, they were not compared with surgical findings or post-mortem dissections [39, 40]. In 2019, Obusez *et al.* evaluated the use of MR imaging of the vessel wall ("VW-MR") to determine the exact location of unruptured paraclinoid aneurysms in relation to DDR but, once again, the study ran into low statistical power and there was no comparison with surgery or necropsy study to verify the findings [41]. Therefore, until now, there is no knowledge of accuracy studies for the diagnostic tests of paraclinoid aneurysms and their relationship with the cavernous sinus. The studies found are series of cases that did not determine sensitivity, specificity, predictive values, and likelihood ratios [24, 37–40, 42–46].

Therefore, the preoperative identification of the distal dural ring and the actual definition of the limits of the roof of the cavernous sinus in relation to paraclinoid aneurysms remains an unresolved problem. This dilemma stimulated the studies of the authors of this chapter to develop more adequate preoperative evaluation protocols and proposed the adequate formatting of 3-tesla MRI studies with sensitivity and specificity sufficiently capable of determining the exact location of these AI in relation to the cavernous sinus, the which allows an effective diagnosis and enables a more adequate, safe, and efficient surgical planning. Next, we will describe the formulation of these protocols of great interest for neuroradiological and neurosurgical practice.

2. Original studies that define the precise anatomical relationship between the intradural and intracavernous compartments applied to the context of paraclinoid aneurysms

2.1 Method based on 3t MR images compared with 3D models, anatomy in cadaveric and microsurgical specimen

This method documented the correlation between the oculomotor nerve and the internal carotid artery, assuming their intersection, visualized in a 3 T magnetic resonance study and confirmed from printed three-dimensional biomodels and microsurgery, as a new anatomical-radiological paradigm that marks the upper limit of the cavernous segment of the internal carotid artery, distinguishing paraclinoid intracranial aneurysms. This is a retrospective study carried out in four stages: anatomical, radiological, 3D printing stage and surgical stage. The internal carotid arteries were dissected in their clinoid topography of 10 cadaveric specimens, totaling 20 cerebral hemispheres. Magnetic resonance images and 3D biomodels of 42 aneurysms from 34 patients were analyzed [47].

Magnetic resonance imaging and MRI angiography were performed in a 3 Tesla (3 T) (Siemens-Skyra Evolve, Erlangen, Germany) and GE (GE Health care, HDXT, Milwaukee, USA) machine using a 32- and 8-channel dedicated skull coil, with the objective of identifying the course of the III nerve when crossing laterally with the ICA, inferring at this point the presence of the carotid-oculomotor membrane and correlating this point to the paraclinoid aneurysm under study (**Figure 3**).

High-resolution images were acquired, following the established protocol, in 2D Coronal T2 Fast Spin Echo (FSE) sequences with thin sections, intracranial arterial magnetic AngioMRI in the 3D TOF technique with and without gadolinium, for vascular analysis. The detailed protocol of imaging studies can be found in [47].

The following structures were analyzed: Identification of the internal carotid artery ICA, identification of the oculomotor nerve in all its extension. Identification of anatomical repairs - Anterior Clinoidal Process (ACP), Ophthalmic Artery (OphA), Optic Nerve (ON), Optical Strut (OS), Diaphragm Sellae (DS); Identification of the paraclinoid aneurysm in the patient under study and the relationships of its neck and dome with the III cranial nerve. The intersection between the internal carotid artery (ICA) and the III nerve was identified on CORONAL T2 / CORONAL FIESTA / volumetric T1 with intravenous contrast and post-gadolinium AXIAL 3D TOF sequences.

According to their relationship with the III nerve, paraclinoid aneurysms were classified as follows: Superior to the superior border of the III nerve, whose neck and dome are located distal to the intersection ICA X ON, in an extracavernous location; at the level of the superior border of the III nerve or in a transitional location (with a part of the aneurysmal neck or dome located superiorly and another part inferiorly to the superior border of the ON in its intersection with the ICA); and inferior to the upper border of the oculomotor nerve, in an intracavernous location, when the aneurysm neck and the dome are located below the ICA x III nerve intersection.

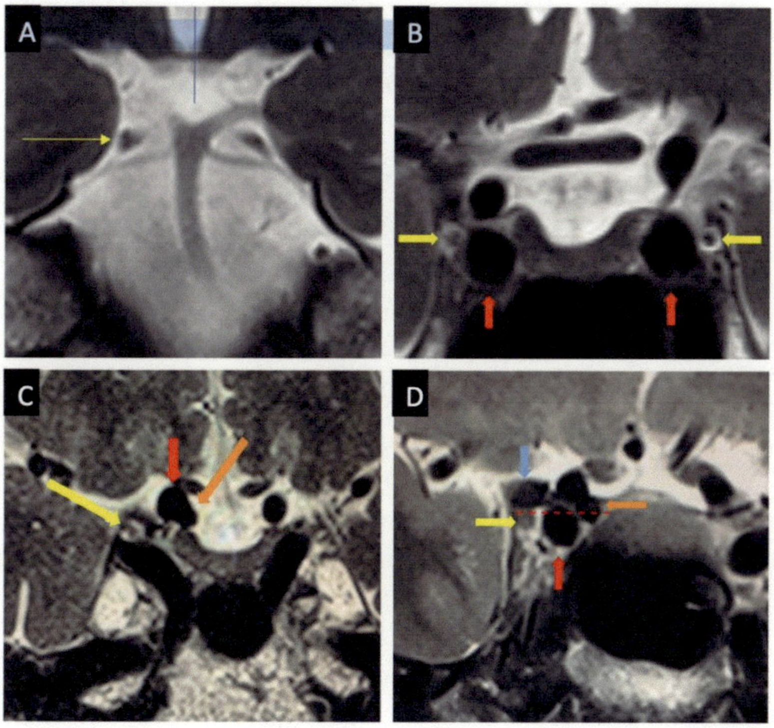

Figure 3.
(A) Bilateral identification of NO on 3 T MRI in T2, coronal sections. In this section, both ONs are contained in the interpeduncular cistern between the posterior cerebral artery, superiorly, and the superior cerebellar artery, inferiorly. We used this cut to begin following ON on its path from the midbrain to the cavernous sinus, in view of the ease with which ON could be identified without a doubt. (B) Location of ON (yellow arrows) and ICA (red arrows) left and right, on 3 T MRI T2 sequence coronal thin slices. Emphasis on the cerebrospinal fluid cistern adjacent to the ON, halo of hypersignal provided by the cerebrospinal fluid, circumcising the ON in the imminence of its entry into the posterior roof of the cavernous sinus, in the topography of the ON triangle. (C) Location of ON (yellow arrow), ICA (red arrow) and left A1 (orange arrow) on 3 T MRI in T2 sequence, axial view. Again, emphasis on the halo provided by the cerebrospinal fluid circumcising the ON, a cistern adjacent to the ON, exactly on the verge of its entry into the posterior roof of the cavernous sinus, within the ON triangle. We used this cistern as a marker to identify cranial nerve III in its path from posterior to anterior, in its transition from the cisternal portion (posterior) to the intracavernous portion (anterior). (D) Identification of ON (yellow arrow) at its intersection with the paraclinoid ICA (red arrow) in the cavernous sinus. The ACP (blue arrow) can be seen just above the NO. The dashed line connecting the upper border of the ON, laterally, to the ICA, medially, is used for evaluation and classification of the AI under study, classified as superior or extracavernous in this image – the entire neck of the aneurysm is found above the upper border of the ON. Caption: ICA – internal carotid artery, NO – oculomotor nerve, ACP – anterior clinoid process, OphA – ophthalmic artery, ON – optic nerve, OS – optic strut, DS – diaphragm sellae, IA – intracranial aneurysm, CSF – cerebrospinal fluid (images kindly provided by Dr. Hugo Doria, MD PhD [47]).

To obtain the 3D model, it was necessary to compile Computed Tomography (CT) and 3-tesla Magnetic Resonance images and computational processing for conversion into STL format (STereoLithography – Stereolithography or triangular pattern language - 3D file of the region of interest). These data were downloaded to the 3D printer, which deposited the chosen material layer by layer, thus forming the desired object on a scale of 140% of the original size for a better visualization of the structures (**Figure 4**).

Of the 34 patients participating in the study, with a total of 42 intracranial aneurysms, 20 patients, totaling 23 aneurysms, underwent intracranial vascular microsurgery for clipping the paraclinoid aneurysm. In the comparative analysis between the

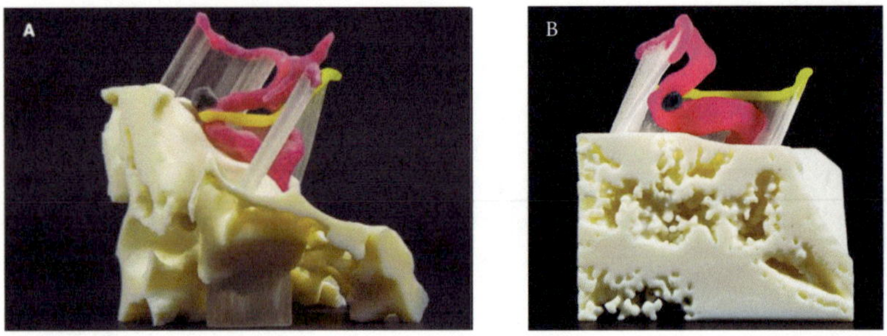

Figure 4.
3D biomodel made from radiological images of patients, showing the structures: ICA – internal carotid artery, printed in red; IA – intracranial aneurysm, printed in black; NO – oculomotor nerve, printed in yellow; bone at the base of the skull, printed in white. In A: evidence of IA classified as extracavernous or greater than the upper limit of the ON at its intersection with the ICA. In B: evidence of IA classified as intracavernous or inferior to the upper limit of the ON at its intersection with the ICA. In transparent acrylic, the supports for supporting the anatomical structures in their exact anatomical positions after three-dimensional printing were printed (images kindly provided by Dr. Hugo Doria, MD PhD [47]).

radiological study and the 3D model of these 42 cases, 40 (95.23%) were considered compatible and of these, 36 (90%) obtained total compatibility in the 3 (neuroradiologist 1 / neuroradiologist 2 / 3D biomodel) evaluations and classifications and 4 (10%) obtained compatibility between 2 of the 3 evaluators (neuroradiologist 1 or neuroradiologist 2 compatible with the 3D biomodel), and the three-dimensional biomodel is the parameter of success in view of its total accuracy and anatomical-radiological reliability (**Figure 5**).

The results together indicate that, in the impossibility of directly identifying the ADP, the identification of the upper limit of the III cranial nerve immediately lateral to the ICA, in all its diameter, and the distance between the III cranial nerve and the ICA can be considered a landmark for delimitation of the roof of the cavernous sinus distinguishing intracavernous ICA and extracavernous ICA since the measurements were close both in the 20 brain hemispheres dissected in 10 anatomical specimens (average distance of 1.19 mm - ranging from 0.6 mm to 1.7 mm) and in the 34 patients studied radiologically (average distance of 1.09 mm - ranging from 0.4 mm to 2.6 mm).

Of the 42 aneurysms studied, twenty-three (54.76%) underwent intracranial vascular microsurgical treatment by clipping, which confirmed the classification of the aneurysm as extracavernous, corroborating the findings in the anatomical specimens and in the radiological analyzes and printed 3D biomodel and indicated that the distance between the III cranial nerve and the ICA can be a landmark for delimiting the ceiling of the cavernous sinus, distinguishing intracavernous ICA and extracavernous ICA.

In summary, in cadaveric specimens, totaling 20 cavernous sinuses studied, we identified that the upper limit of the cavernous sinus is determined by the carotid-oculomotor membrane (COMM), which closely correlates to the intersection between the internal carotid artery and the oculomotor nerve, crossing it, transversely across its entire diameter.

Corroborating the anatomical step, we identified the intersection between the oculomotor nerve and the internal carotid artery in 3 Tesla brain magnetic resonance images of 42 aneurysms. The intersection between the oculomotor nerve and the internal carotid artery was established as a new anatomical-radiological landmark for paraclinoid aneurysms in terms of the carotid segment in which they are contained, intra or extracavernous; The 3D biomodel confirmed the radiological precision for the

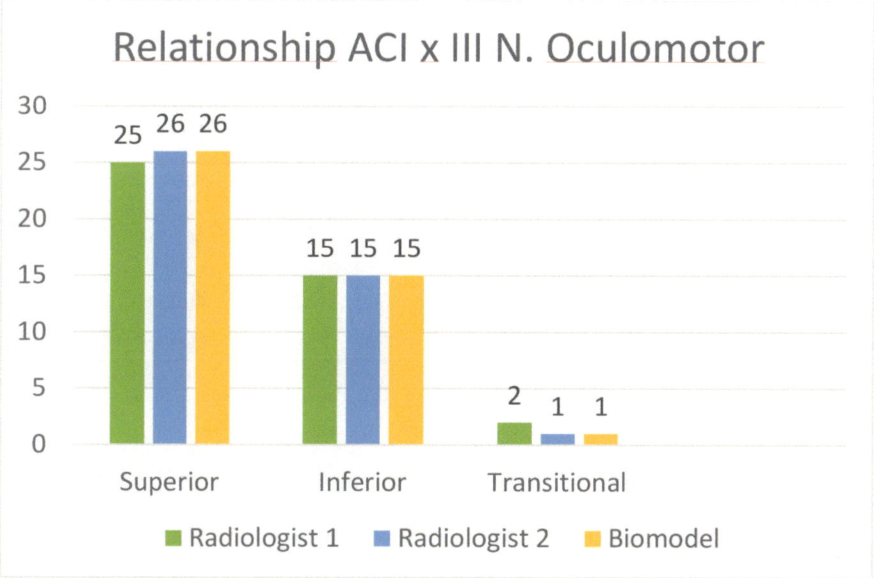

Figure 5.
Comparison between the classification of paraclinoidal aneurysms by the two neuroradiologists, in a blind and independent manner, and the classification by the printed three-dimensional biomodel. The radiologists, blindly and independently, classified the aneurysms according to their relationship between the aneurysmal neck and the intersection between the ON and the ICA, as superior, transitional, or inferior to the superior limit of the III cranial nerve, while the author of the work classified the aneurysms based on the processing of CT, MR and Angio RM 3 Tesla images and analysis of the three-dimensional biomodel from the 3D printing (Modification and Publication authorized by Dr. Hugo Doria, MD PhD [47]).

exact location of the paraclinoid aneurysms, showing high compatibility for the location of the analyzed paraclinoid aneurysms. The surgical procedure performed in 23 aneurysms confirmed this legend and allows formulating a new paradigm for classifying paraclinoid aneurysms, between: extracavernous or superior, intracavernous, or inferior, or transitional in the preoperative stage, thus avoiding surgical exploration and its associated risks.

2.2 Method based on 3t MR images compared with microsurgical anatomy

This is a cross-sectional clinical study of diagnostic accuracy that analyzed a prospective cohort of 20 patients totaling 25 paraclinoid aneurysms in a single hospital center in São Paulo in the period between 2014 and 2018 [48].

The patients underwent Cerebral Angiography with Digital Subtraction, which characterized the sample with 10 cavernous and 15 non-cavernous aneurysms, as shown in the table below (**Table 1**).

The same sample of patients underwent a 3-tesla MRI study with the specific protocol detailed in [48]. The following structures were analyzed: distal dural ring (DDA); proximal dural ring (PDR); Anterior Clinoid Process (ACP), ICA, Ophthalmic Artery (OphA), Optic Nerve (ON), Optic Strut (OS), Diaphragm Sellae (DS); identification of the paraclinoid aneurysm and the relationships of its neck and dome with adjacent structures. DDR has been identified as the reflection of the dura mater surrounding the ICA as it leaves the roof of the cavernous sinus. It is contained in a curved dural plane that projects inferomedially between the median crest of the

	Localization			
Variable	**General (25)**	**Cavernous (10)**	**Not Cavernous (15)**	*P Value*
Age (average ± DP)	51,4 ± 11,5	48,5 ± 13,8	53,3 ± 9,7	0,313
Feminine Gender	24 (96)	10 (100)	14 (93,3)	1000
Size (median e quartiles)	5,0 (4,0 – 5,5)	5,0 (3,0 – 5,3)	5,0 (4,0 – 6,0)	0,511
Guidance				0,322
Superior	7 (28,0)	2 (20,0)	5 (33,3)	
Medial	15 (60,0)	7 (70,0)	8 (53,3)	
Lateral	2 (8,0)	0 (0,0)	2 (13,3)	
Inferior	1 (4,0)	1 (10,0)	0 (0,0)	

Data presented as n (%) unless specified. DP (standard deviation)

Table 1.
Characterization of the sample according to age and gender of patients and size and location of aneurysms, according to Kristh et al [20].

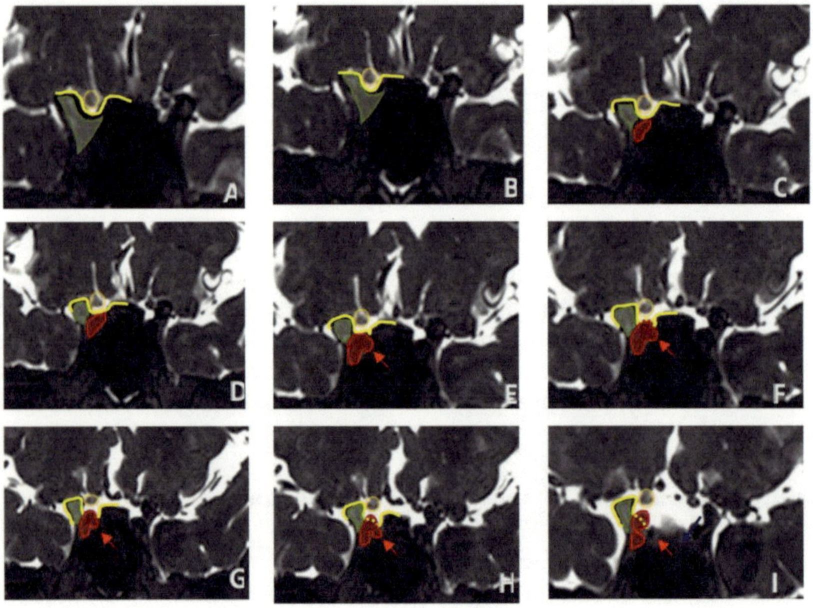

Figure 6.
3-T MRI in T2-weighted turbo-spin sequence in the coronal plane (anterior to posterior, from "A" to "I", respectively) according to the protocol of the present study, demonstrating the anatomo-radiological markers of the paraclinoid region. Note that the optic strut (OS) is identified on MRI as the shade in green and a paraclinoid aneurysm on the right is considered transitional – note in "I", blue arrow, how the most posterior portion of the aneurysm projects into the subarachnoid space. ACP and OS, green; ON, golden; ICA, anterior loop of the internal carotid artery – "C" to "H", red; ICA, cavernous internal carotid artery, horizontal segment – "I"; Aneurysm – "E" to "I", red arrow (adapted and published with permission of Sergio Tadeu Fernandes, MD PhD).

superior surface of the PDA and the diaphragm sellae [39, 40, 42, 49–51]. The DDR also extends infero-posteriorly between the floor of the optic canal and the posterior part of the roof of the cavernous sinus as illustrated in **Figures 6** and 7.

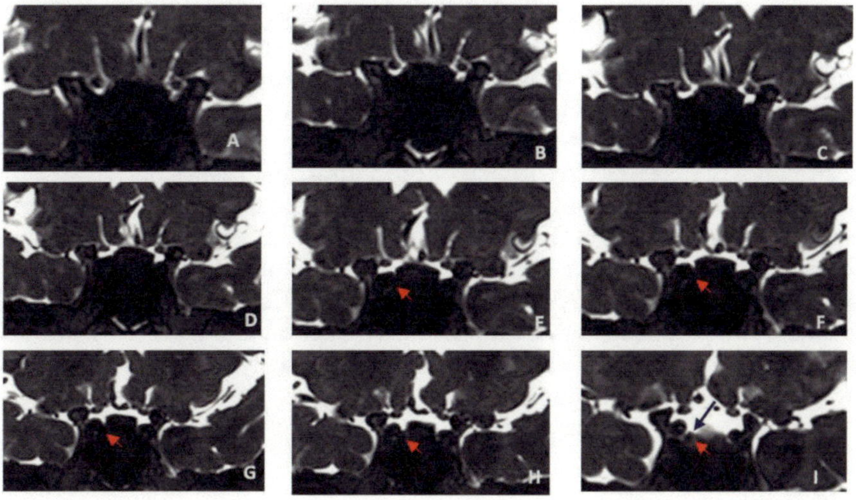

Figure 7.
Removed markers from the previous figure to exercise the identification of structures of interest. Paraclinoid aneurysm on the right is considered transitional – note on "I", blue arrow, how the most posterior portion of the aneurysm projects into the subarachnoid space – aneurysm – "E" to "I", red arrow (adapted and published with permission of Sergio Tadeu Fernandes, MD PhD).

Classification		Surgery		Total
		Cavernous	Not Cavernous	
MRI	Cavernous	9 (36,0)	2 (8,0)	11 (44,4)
	Not Cavernous	1 (4,0)	13 (52,0)	14 (56,0)
	Total	10 (40)	15 (60)	25 (100)

Data presented as n (% of total). Kappa: 0.754, p < 0.001. MRI: magnetic resonance imaging

Table 2.
Agreement analysis between MRI and surgery.

After analysis by the neuroradiologist, the following results were obtained: 11 (44.4%) were classified as intracavernous, 1 (4%) as transitional and 13 (52%) as intradural. Finally, the patients underwent microsurgical treatment of AI clipping. Of the 25 aneurysms analyzed during the microsurgical procedure and exploration of the paraclinoid region, 10 (40%) were classified as intracavernous, 2 (8%) as transitional and 13 (52%) as intradural. The comparative analysis of these data can be seen in **Table 2**.

Data processing showed that the accuracy of magnetic resonance imaging in terms of the intracavernous or intradural location of the aneurysm, with the intraoperative finding as the gold standard and the characteristic "presence of disease" or "positive test" for non-cavernous aneurysm, found sensitivity of 86.7% (95% CI, 59.5–98.3), specificity of 90.0 (95% CI, 55.5–99.8), positive and negative likelihood ratios of 8.7 (CI 95%, 1.3–56.2) and 0.15 (95% CI, 0.04–0.6), respectively, and positive and negative predictive values of 92.9 (95% CI, 66.1–99.8) and 81.8 (95% CI, 48.2–97.7), respectively. The inter-observer agreement by Cohen's Kappa method was almost perfect ($\kappa = 0.901$; $p < 0.001$; 95% CI, 0.71–1.00) between MRI and surgical procedure findings. The diagnostic test in individuals with no history of SAH had a sensitivity of 92.3% and specificity of 100%. In this circumstance, the 100% specificity demonstrates the superiority of MRI when the aneurysm is intracavernous, that is, it is a method free of false negatives and can be considered the gold standard in ruling out the presence of disease (transitional or intradural aneurysm).

Transferring the issue to daily practice, it can be stated that, when considering the preoperative MRI result in the decision-making process for conservative treatment of paraclinoid aneurysms with no history of SAH, it is likely that all aneurysms considered cavernous, fact they are. The practical significance of these findings is that absolutely all patients eligible for preventive treatment of SAH (transitional or intradural aneurysms) will be so diagnosed and, eventually, only 1 in 10 of treated cases would not need treatment (cavernous aneurysms – false negatives).

3. Conclusion

MRI acquisition protocols demonstrated here are able to accurately define aneurysms in the paraclinoid region in terms of their location in relation to the cavernous sinus and, therefore, provides more appropriate and reliable recommendations for the management of paraclinoid aneurysms smaller than 10 mm regarding conservative or interventional (coiling or clipping) treatment options.

Acknowledgements

The authors would like to thank all collaborators of HTEJZ - SPDM, on behalf of its CEO, Otávio Monteiro Becker Jr., MD, PhD.

Conflict of interest

The authors declare no conflict of interest.

Author details

Sérgio Tadeu Fernandes[1]*, Hugo Leonardo Dória-Netto[2] and Edson Bernaldino Neto[3]

1 Department of Vascular Neurosurgery at the Hospital de Transplantes Euryclides de Jesus Zerbini-SPDM, São Paulo, Brazil

2 Vascular Neurosurgeon at the Hospital de Transplantes Euryclides de Jesus Zerbini - SPDM, Vascular Neurosurgeon at the São Paulo Hospital – UNIFESP, São Paulo, Brazil

3 Neurosurgeon Member of the Brazilian Society of Neurosurgery, Fellowship of Vascular Neurosurgery at the Hospital de Transplantes Euryclides de Jesus Zerbini-SPDM, São Paulo, Brazil

*Address all correspondence to: s_tadeu@outlook.com

References

[1] Etminan N, Dreier R, Buchholz BA, Beseoglu K, Bruckner P, Matzenauer C, et al. Age of collagen in intracranial saccular aneurysms. Stroke. 2014;**45**(6):1757-1763

[2] Lasheras JC. The Biomechanics of arterial. Aneurysms. 2006;**39**:293-319 Available from: https://www.annualreviews.org/doi/abs/10.1146/annurev.fluid.39.050905.110128

[3] Frösen J. Smooth muscle cells and the formation, degeneration, and rupture of saccular intracranial aneurysm wall--a review of current pathophysiological knowledge. Translational Stroke Research. 2014;**5**(3):347-356 Available from: https://pubmed.ncbi.nlm.nih.gov/24683005/

[4] Frösen J, Tulamo R, Paetau A, Laaksamo E, Korja M, Laakso A, et al. Saccular intracranial aneurysm: Pathology and mechanisms. Acta Neuropathologica. 2012;**12386**(6):773-786

[5] Kurki MI, Häkkinen SK, Frösen J, Tulamo R, von Und Z, Fraunberg M, et al. Upregulated signaling pathways in ruptured human saccular intracranial aneurysm wall: An emerging regulative role of toll-like receptor signaling and nuclear factor-κB, hypoxia-inducible factor-1A, and ETS transcription factors. Neurosurgery. 2011;**68**(6):1667-1675

[6] Starke R, Chalouhi N, Ali M, Jabbour P, Tjoumakaris S, Gonzalez L, et al. The role of oxidative stress in cerebral aneurysm formation and rupture. Current Neurovascular Research. 2013;**10**(3):247-255

[7] Vega C, Kwoon J, v., Lavine SD. Intracranial aneurysms: Current evidence and clinical practice. American Family Physician. 2002;**66**(4):601-608

[8] Etminan N, Rinkel GJ. Unruptured intracranial aneurysms: Development, rupture and preventive management. Nature Reviews. Neurology. 2016: dez 1212):699-713.

[9] Chalouhi N, Hoh BL, Hasan D. Review of cerebral aneurysm formation, growth, and rupture. Stroke. 2013;**44**(12):3613-3622

[10] Rhoton AL. The supratentorial arteries. Neurosurgery. 2002;**51**(4):53-120

[11] Rhoton AL. The cavernous sinus, the cavernous venous plexus, and the carotid collar. Neurosurgery. 2002;**51**(4):375-410

[12] Rhoton AL. Aneurysms. Neurosurgery. 2002;**51**(4):121-158

[13] Vlak MHM, Algra A, Brandenburg R, Rinkel GJE. Prevalence of unruptured intracranial aneurysms, with emphasis on sex, age, comorbidity, country, and time period: A systematic review and meta-analysis. Lancet Neurology. 2011;**10**(7):626-636

[14] Chalouhi N, Ali MS, Jabbour PM, Tjoumakaris SI, Gonzalez LF, Rosenwasser RH, et al. Biology of intracranial aneurysms: Role of inflammation. Journal of Cerebral Blood Flow and Metabolism. 2012;**3276**(9):1659-1676

[15] Micieli JA, Newman NJ, Barrow DL, Biousse V. Intracranial aneurysms of neuro-ophthalmologic relevance. Journal of Neuro-Ophthalmology. 2017;**37**(4):421-439

[16] Frösen J, Piippo A, Paetau A, Kangasniemi M, Niemelä M, Hernesniemi J, et al. Remodeling of saccular cerebral artery aneurysm wall is associated with rupture: Histological analysis of 24 unruptured and 42 ruptured cases. Stroke. 2004;**35**(10):2287-2293

[17] Munarriz PM, Gómez PA, Paredes I, Castaño-Leon AM, Cepeda S, Lagares A. Basic principles of hemodynamics and cerebral aneurysms. World Neurosurgery;**2016**(88):311-319

[18] Drake CG, Vanderlinden RG, Amacher AL. Carotid-ophthalmic aneurysms. Journal of Neurosurgery. 1968;**29**(1):24-31

[19] Kim JM, Romano A, Sanan A, van Loveren HR, Keller JT. Microsurgical anatomic features and nomenclature of the paraclinoid region. Neurosurgery. 2000;**46**(3):670-682

[20] Krisht AF, Hsu SPC. Paraclinoid Aneurysms: Part IV-Medial Aneurysms. 2020. Available from: www.contempneurosurg.com

[21] Bouthillier A, van Loveren HR, Keller JT. Segments of the internal carotid artery: A new classification. Neurosurgery. 1996;**38**(3):425-433

[22] Kobayashi S, Kyoshima K, Gibo H, Hegde SA, Takemae T, Sugita K. Carotid cave aneurysms of the internal carotid artery. Journal of Neurosurgery. 1989;**70**(2):216-221

[23] Joo W, Funaki T, Yoshioka F, Rhoton AL. Microsurgical anatomy of the carotid cave. Neurosurgery. 2012;**70**(2)

[24] Gonzalez LF, Walker MT, Zabramski JM, Partovi S, Wallace RC, Spetzler RF, et al. Distinction between paraclinoid and cavernous sinus aneurysms with computed tomographic angiography. Neurosurgery. 2003;**52**(5):1131-1139 Available from: https://utsouthwestern.pure.elsevier.com/en/publications/distinction-between-paraclinoid-and-cavernous-sinus-aneurysms-wit

[25] Brown B, Hanel RA. Endovascular management of cavernous and paraclinoid aneurysms. Neurosurgery Clinical North America. 2014;**25**(3):415-424. Available from: https://pubmed.ncbi.nlm.nih.gov/24994081/

[26] Sengupta RP, Gryspeerdt GL, Hankinson J. Carotid-ophthalmic aneurysms. Journal of Neurological Neurosurgery Psychiatry. 2022;**39**(9):837-853 Available from: https://pubmed.ncbi.nlm.nih.gov/993805/

[27] Hoh BL, Carter BS, Budzik RF, Putman CM, Ogilvy CS. Results after surgical and endovascular treatment of paraclinoid aneurysms by a combined neurovascular team. Neurosurgery. 2001;**48**(1):78-90 Available from: https://pubmed.ncbi.nlm.nih.gov/11152364/

[28] Roy D, Raymond J, Bouthillier A, Bojanowski MW, Moumdjian R, L'Espérance G. Endovascular treatment of ophthalmic segment aneurysms with Guglielmi detachable coils. AJNR American Journal of Neuroradiology. 2001;**18**(2):1207-1215 Available from: https://europepmc.org/articles/PMC8338007

[29] Colen TW, Wang LC, Ghodke B, Cohen WA, Hollingworth W, Anzai Y et al. Effectiveness of MDCT Angiography for the Detection of Intracranial Aneurysms in Patients with Nontraumatic Subarachnoid Hemorrhage. 2007. Available from: www.ajronline.org

[30] Mayberg MR, Batjer HH, Dacey R, Diringer M, Haley EC, Heros RC, et al. Guidelines for the management of aneurysmal subarachnoid hemorrhage. A statement for healthcare professionals from a special writing group of the Stroke Council, American Heart Association. Stroke. 1994;**25**(11):2315-2328 Available from: https://pubmed.ncbi.nlm.nih.gov/7974568/

[31] Villablanca JP, Achiriolaie A, Hooshi P, Martin N, Duckwiler G, Jahan R, et al. Aneurysms of the posterior circulation: Detection and treatment planning using volume-rendered three-dimensional helical computerized tomography angiography. Journal of Neurosurgery. 2005;**103**(6):1018-1026 Available from: https://pubmed.ncbi.nlm.nih.gov/16381188/

[32] Lehto H, Kivisaari R, Niemelä M, Dashti R, Elsharkawy A, Harati A, et al. Seventy aneurysms of the posterior inferior cerebellar artery: Anatomical features and value of computed tomography angiography in microneurosurgery. World Neurosurgery 2014 dez;**82**(6):1106-1112

[33] Gibo H, Lenkey C, Rhoton AL. Microsurgical anatomy of the supraclinoid portion of the internal carotid artery. Journal of Neurosurgery. 1981;**55**(4):560-574

[34] Renn WH, Rhoton AL. Microsurgical anatomy of the sellar region. Journal of Neurosurgery. 1975;**43**(3):288-298

[35] Nishio S, Matsushima T, Fukui M, Sawada K, Kitamura K. Microsurgical anatomy around the origin of the ophthalmic artery with reference to contralateral pterional surgical approach to the carotid-ophthalmic aneurysm. Acta Neurochirurgica. 1985;**76**(3):82-89

[36] Oikawa S, Kyoshima K, Kobayashi S. Surgical anatomy of the juxta-dural ring area. Journal of Neurosurgery. 1998;**89**(2):250-254

[37] Murayama Y, Sakumura K, Satoh K, Nagahiro S. Identification of the carotid artery dural ring by using three-dimensional computerized tomography angiography. Journal of Neurosurgery. 2001;**95**(3):533-536

[38] Hashimoto K, Nozaki K, Hashimoto N. Optic strut as a radiographic landmark in evaluating neck location of a paraclinoid aneurysm. Neurosurgery. 2006;**59**(4):880-885

[39] Thines L, Gauvrit JY, Leclerc X, le Gars D, Delmaire C, Pruvo JP, et al. Usefulness of MR imaging for the assessment of nonophthalmic paraclinoid aneurysms. American Journal of Neuroradiology. 2008;**29**(1):125-129

[40] Thines L, Seon KL, Dehdashti AR, Agid R, Willinsky RA, Wallace CM, et al. Direct imaging of the distal dural ring and paraclinoid internal carotid artery aneurysms with high-resolution T2 turbo-spin echo technique at 3-T magnetic resonance imaging. Neurosurgery. 2009;**64**(6):1059-1064

[41] Obusez EC, Jones SE, Mandell D, Bullen J, Gonzalez F, Hui FK. Feasibility of vessel wall imaging in assessing unruptured paraclinoid aneurysms: Clinical observations and preliminary experience. Journal of Clinical Neuroscience. 2019;**61**:59-65

[42] Lee N, Jung JY, Huh SK, Kim DJ, Kim DI, Kim J. Distinction between Intradural and extradural aneurysms involving the Paraclinoid internal carotid artery with T2-weighted three-dimensional fast spin-Echo magnetic resonance imaging. Journal of Korean Neurosurgery Society. 2022;**47**(6):437-441. Available from: http://www.ncbi.nlm.nih.gov/pubmed/20617089

[43] Eddleman CS, Hurley MC, Bendok BR, Batjer HH. Cavernous carotid aneurysms: To treat or not to treat? Neurosurgical Focus. 2009;**26**(5):1-20

[44] Ito K, Hongo K, Kakizawa Y, Kobayashi S, Partovi S, Spetzler RF, et al. Three-dimensional contrast medium-enhanced computed tomographic cisternography for preoperative evaluation of surgical anatomy of intradural paraclinoid aneurysms of the internal carotid artery: Technical note. Neurosurgery. 2002;**51**(4):1089-1093

[45] Tsuboi T, Tokunaga K, Shingo T, Itoh T, Mandai S, Kinugasa K, et al. Differentiation between intradural and extradural locations of juxta-dural ring aneurysms by using contrast-enhanced 3-dimensional time-of-flight magnetic resonance angiography. Surgical Neurology. 2007;**67**(4):381-387

[46] Thines L, Delmaire C, le Gars D, Pruvo JP, Lejeune JP, Lehmann P, et al. MRI location of the distal dural ring plane: Anatomoradiological study and application to paraclinoid carotid artery aneurysms. European Radiology. 2006;**16**(2):479-488

[47] Doria-Netto HL, Campos CM, Marussi VH, Campos-Filho JM, Faber J, Lawton MT, et al. The Intersection Between the Oculomotor Nerve and the Internal Carotid Artery to Distinguish Extracavernous and Intracavernous Paraclinoid Aneurysms Using Anatomic Dissections-A New 3T Magnetic Resonance Imaging Protocol Confirmed by Three-Dimensionally Printed Biomodels. World Neurosurgery. 2022;**167**:e475-e506 Available from: https://pubmed.ncbi.nlm.nih.gov/35970294/

[48] Fernandes ST, Doria-Netto HL, Alves RV, Lapate RL, Ferreira NPFD, Teixeira MJ, et al. The diagnostic accuracy of MRI in determining the relations between paraclinoid aneurysms and the cavernous sinus. Neuroradiology. 2022;**64**(6):1175 Available from: /pmc/articles/PMC9117373/

[49] Seoane E, Rhoton AL, de Oliveira E. Microsurgical anatomy of the dural collar (carotid collar) and rings around the clinoid segment of the internal carotid artery. Neurosurgery. 1998;**42**(4):869-886

[50] de Jesús O, Sekhar LN, Riedel CJ. Clinoid and paraclinoid aneurysms: Surgical anatomy, operative techniques, and outcome. Surgical Neurology. 1999;**51**(5):477-488

[51] Johnston SC, Wilson CB, Halbach V, Higashida RT, Dowd CF, MW MD, et al. Endovascular and surgical treatment of unruptured cerebral aneurysms: Comparison of risks. Annals of Neurology. 2000;**48**(1):11-19

Chapter 2

Aneurysmal Subarachnoid Hemorrhage and Early Brain Injury: A New Pathophysiological Perspective

Guilherme Nascimento de Morais and Salomón Rojas

Abstract

Non-traumatic subarachnoid hemorrhage is a devastating neurological emergency, the main cause of which is aneurysmal rupture. The treatment of the aneurysm, whether microsurgical or endovascular, is essential for the recovery of these patients, however, a series of pathophysiological events in the days following the bleeding cause great damage to the brain tissue. For many years efforts have been focused on the prevention and treatment of cerebral vasospasm, which is believed to be the cause of late cerebral ischemia. However, new pathophysiological perspectives point to a series of events that begin immediately after bleeding, known as early brain injury, mainly involving brain microvascular dysfunction, cortical spreading depolarizations and neuroinflammation, which we discuss below.

Keywords: subarachnoid hemorrhage, early brain injury, microvascular dysfunction, cortical spreading depolarizations, neuroinflammation

1. Introduction

Non-traumatic subarachnoid hemorrhage is a devastating neurological emergency, resulting from the rupture of cerebral aneurysms in most cases. It accounts for about 5–7% of strokes each year, with high morbidity and mortality [1]. Approximately 10% of patients die before receiving medical care [2]. This occurs due to a metabolic collapse caused by the sudden and sustained increase in intracranial pressure (ICP), reducing cerebral perfusion and causing global cerebral ischemia. For those who do receive medical care, about 25% die in the first 24 to 72 hours, with the level of consciousness, hemorrhage volume and neurological deficits on admission being determinants for the prognosis. In this time window, a series of pathophysiological events are known as early brain injury (EBI) [3], including neuroinflammation, microvascular dysfunction and cortical spreading depolarizations (SD), which recent studies point out as main events related to worse prognosis in aneurysmal subarachnoid hemorrhage (SAH). Survivors of this period are still subject to secondary brain injuries resulting from vasospasm of medium and large caliber intracranial arteries, in up to 70% of patients, and even delayed cerebral ischemia (DCI), in 30% of cases [1]. Typically, vasospasm has its highest incidence between the third and fourteenth day after the ictus, occurring due to the imbalance between vasodilator and vasoconstrictor factors in the subarachnoid space, including an increase in the concentration of bilirubin oxidation products, formed from hemoglobin [4]. New focal neurological deficits or a two-point drop on the Glasgow Coma Scale (GCS), within an hour, in turn characterizes DCI [5].

For many years, it was believed that the worst neurocognitive outcomes of SAH occurred as a result of distal hypoperfusion caused by vasospasm of the cerebral arteries, therefore, efforts were focused on the treatment of this entity [6]. Although not yet fully elucidated, the pathogenesis of vasospasm is correlated with high concentrations of Endothelin-1 (ET-1) in the cerebrospinal fluid (CSF). This peptide, made up of 21 amino acids, synthesized by the endothelium, has a potent vasoconstrictor action, also present in other non-neurological pathologies, such as infectious diseases, pulmonary arterial hypertension and neoplasms. In the brain, ET-1 activates $ET\text{-}_A$ receptors, leading to increased cellular calcium influx into smooth muscle, resulting in vasoconstriction [7]. Clazosentan, a highly selective ET-A receptor antagonist, has studied as a treatment for vasospasm and DCI. A double-blind, randomized, phase 2 study of 413 patients showed a reduction in the incidence of angiographic vasospasm from 66% in the placebo group to 23% in the control group (65% risk reduction - 95% CI, $P < 0.0001$) [8], however, the benefit in morbidity and mortality related to vasospasm, evaluating the functional outcome in patients was not confirmed by the subsequent phase 3 study [9]. These results served as a turning point in the field of post-SAH brain injuries, highlighting the importance of researching other pathophysiological mechanisms [10]. From then on, a series of studies were concerned with investigating the mechanisms in the early stage of the disease, with great advances in EBI, which is the focus of the study in this chapter.

2. EBI mechanisms

Brain damage in SAH begins immediately after bleeding. A sudden increase in ICP, caused by intracranial bleeding, causes a reduction in cerebral perfusion and impairment of brain hemodynamics, impairing the mechanisms of self-regulation of brain blood flow, which results in ischemia of the brain tissue, triggering a series of events called "ischemic cascade" [11]. During oxygen and glucose deprivation, there is a reduction in the production of adenosine triphosphate (ATP) and consequent reduction in the activity of Na^+/K^+-ATPase, with loss of cellular ionic homeostasis, with an increase in the concentration of intracellular Na^+ and cytotoxic edema. The exit of K^+ from neurons and the entry of Na^+ into the cytoplasm cause cell depolarization. Depolarized neurons are unable to restore their action potentials and die within minutes as a result of energy collapse and a cycle of loss of ionic homeostasis, cytotoxic edema, proteolysis and disintegration of cell membranes [12]. In addition, anaerobic metabolism in areas of greater energy susceptibility generates tissue acidosis, with breakdown of the blood-brain barrier (BBB) and dilation of pre-capillary arterioles, generating vasogenic edema, increased brain volume and ICP, reduced brain perfusion pressure and encephalic hemodynamic collapse.

Concomitantly to this, after bleeding, platelets activated, leading to platelet aggregation and formation of microthrombosis in the microcirculation (which may contain

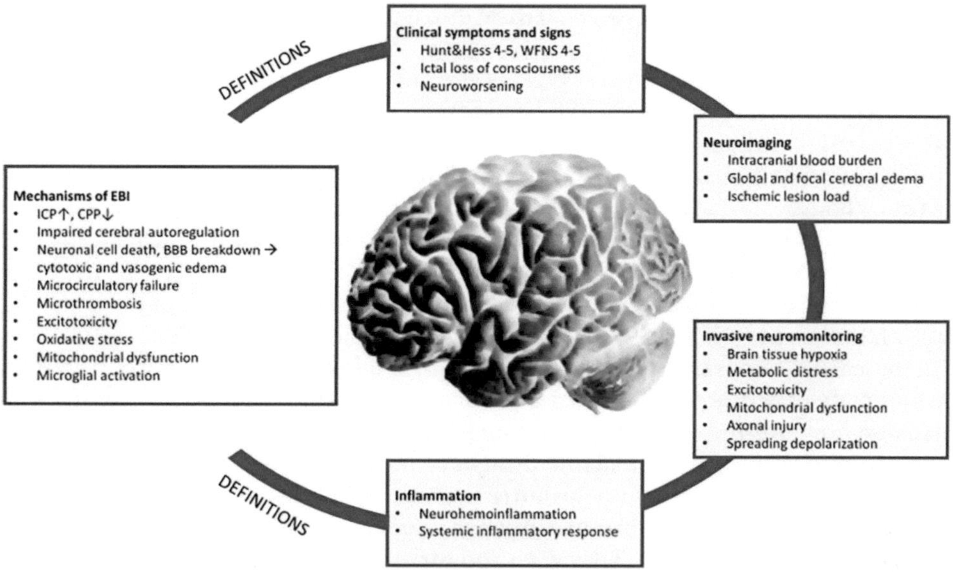

Figure 1.
Complex pathophysiological mechanisms that contribute to EBI after SAH. Reprinted from Rass et al., current neurology and neuroscience, 2019 [11].

red blood cells and white blood cells in their composition). This causes increased cerebrovascular resistance and perfusion impairment. The reduction in cerebral flow generates blood stasis and the propagation of intravascular microthrombosis, perpetuating the process of tissue ischemia [13].

In addition to perfusion impairment, "non-ischemic" mechanisms are related to EBI, such as energy/mitochondrial dysfunction caused by SD and, finally, a complex and wide range of reactions caused by microglial activation, culminating in neurinflammation (**Figure 1**) [11].

2.1 Microvascular dysfunction

The brain is a high compliance organ, and it is estimated that cerebral vascular resistance is largely regulated by precapillary arterioles, with a central role in the control of brain hemodynamics. Angiographic vasospasm, observed in up to 70% of patients with SAH, refers to a reduction in the caliber of large vessels, not being correlated in the same proportion to brain tissue ischemia, since the incidence of DCI is observed in half of patients with vasospasm angiographic and occurs even in patients without vasospasm [14]. Such evidence suggests the increasing participation of microvascular dysfunction in brain damage.

At this moment, the only drug that has shown to be beneficial in reducing DCI has been the calcium channel blocker nimodipine. It has no significant effect on vasospasm; however, it inhibits vasoconstriction at the level of precapillary arterioles, suggesting that targeting microvascular dysfunction can improve results in SAH [15]. Some experimental studies with animal models of SAH have investigated microvascular reactivity with direct observation of vessels *in vivo*, as well as the behavior of pial arterioles against vasoactive agents, including adenosine, acetylcholine, carbon dioxide and nitric oxide (NO). In rodents, great damage to microvascular reactivity was observed in the face of these interventions [16, 17].

Another aspect of the microvasculature dysfunction involved in the pathogenesis of cerebral ischemia in SAH is microthrombosis. It is commonly found throughout the brain after SAH, with a greater presence in areas of arteriolar constriction [18] in a pattern called "string of pearls." The main findings of the study by Friedrich et al., with a model of SAH in rodents, are that more than 70% of the arterioles derived from the middle cerebral artery (MCA) presented "string of pearls" constrictions in the first 3 hours after SAH and that these constrictions persisted for at least 3 days after the hemorrhage, suggesting that the vessels become spastic. The arteriolar diameter was reduced by up to 50% and the more constricted the arterioles were, the more often the vessel lumen was occluded by microthrombosis (30% of all spastic vessels). Small reductions in arteriolar diameter can significantly reduce blood flow with increasing cerebral vascular resistance (Poiseuille's law) and microthrombosis can completely disrupt microperfusion, explaining the severe early and cerebral perfusion pressure-independent reduction in cerebral blood flow after SAH [17].

In addition to the mechanical impairment of obstructing blood flow, activation of the coagulation cascade and neuroinflammation are closely linked to each other through a process known as thromboinflammation. A sequence of events that include endothelial adhesion, platelet activation and inflammation, culminate in microthrombosis, ischemia, vasogenic edema and EBI [19]. Platelets amplify the inflammatory cascade. Once activated, platelets display P-selectin and release cytokines that promote leukocyte adhesion and transmigration at sites of platelet deposition. Neutrophils also release factors that promote platelet activation. Activated platelets and inflammatory cells contribute to endothelial rupture, perpetuating the cycle of microthrombosis and inflammation, even far from the site of aneurysm rupture [20]. A study involving 127 patients evaluated platelet activation through the maximum amplitude of thromboelastography (TEG) and inflammation through serum levels of C-reactive protein (CRP) and percentage of neutrophils in venous blood, collected at 0–24, 24–48 and 48–72 hours after aneurysm rupture. They found that patients with high-grade SAH (by Hunt-Hess, NIHSS and GCS scales) had significant elevations in platelet activation and inflammation compared to patients with less severely affected SAH (Hunt-Hess 1–3). Furthermore, there was a "dose-response" effect with incremental increase in platelet activation and inflammation as the Hunt-Hess grade and EBI worsened. Even after controlling for other factors, platelet activation was independently associated with EBI [20].

SAH also generates an imbalance of vasoactive substances, both endogenous vasoconstrictors, such as ET-1, and vasodilators, such as NO [21]. Activated leukocytes in the CSF of patients with SAH synthesize and release ET-1, causing arterial vasoconstriction. As mentioned above, clazosentan, a selective endothelin $ET\text{-}_A$ receptor antagonist was able to reduce angiographic vasospasm [9]. The benefits of this intervention, although uncertain so far with the publication of CONSCIUS-2, are still extensively studied, and another phase 3 study (REACT) is underway, which is intended to assess its efficacy and safety [22]. Japan is the first country where its use approved for the prevention of vasospasm, cerebral infarction related to vasospasm and symptoms of cerebral ischemia after SAH [23].

On the other hand, NO is capable of inducing cyclic guanosine monophosphate (cGMP) mediated vasodilation, in addition to being involved in the post-SAH inflammatory response. In vascular endothelial cells, in the presence of oxygen, the nitrogenous guanidino terminal of L-arginine produces the gaseous free radical, NO and L-citrulline in a process catalyzed by the enzyme nitric oxide synthase (NOS). NO crosses the space of the endothelium to the vascular smooth muscle and directly stimulates the soluble guanylate cyclase enzyme and the consequent formation of intracellular cGMP, resulting in the relaxation of vascular smooth muscle cells. Constant levels of NO keep the arteriolar diameter under normal conditions and prevent platelet and leukocyte activation [24, 25]. In the brain, NO production is mainly provided by neural NOS (nNOS) and endothelial NOS (eNOS). In systemic inflammatory processes its synthesis is mediated by inducible NOS (iNOS). Immediately after bleeding, different mechanisms result in reduced NO bioavailability, such as reduced synthesis, uncoupling of eNOS, endothelial damage, increase in NOS inhibitors (dimethylarginine) and NO sequestration by reactive oxygen species [24]. In the inflammatory response, the upregulation of iNOS by microglia and astrocytes can generate increased levels of NO, inflammation and cytotoxicity by distant microvascular uncoupling. This supports the hypothesis that NO can regulate both microvascular function and neuroinflammation [21].

Attempts to restore NO production balance have been effective in experimental models. Drugs such as L-arginine and S-nitrosoglutathione have shown efficacy in improving outcome after SAH in animal models, but have been associated with drops in systemic blood pressure. However, inhaled NO has limited effects on systemic blood pressure and has been shown, in rodents, to reduce the number and severity of microvascular constrictions with subsequent reduction in mortality and improvement in outcomes. In patients with SAH, NO donors, including sodium nitroprusside and transdermal nitroglycerin, have been used. Some studies have shown promise, however, they are underpowered and side effects of systemic hypotension, headache and rebound hypertension limit routine use [26].

Other therapeutic strategies sought to modulate NO production by interfering with microvascular relaxation in other ways. Phosphodiesterase V (PDE-V) is a regulator that inhibits vascular smooth muscle cell relaxation and subsequent vasodilation. PDE-V inhibition using sildenafil has shown promising results in experimental SAH [27]. Another medication with similar action, the phosphodiesterase III (PDE-III) inhibitor milrinone, showed some effectiveness in reducing vasospasm, with a reduction in the need for endovascular angioplasty and improved results [28]. In addition to PDE inhibitors, magnesium sulfate has shown promise in experimental SAH, with reduction of infarct areas, reversal of vasospasm and improvement of cerebral perfusion based on its ability to promote relaxation of vascular smooth muscle cells [29].

2.2 Cortical spreading depolarizations (SD)

SD was discovered in animals by the Brazilian neurophysiologist Aristides Leão. He suggested that SD is involved in both migraine aura and cerebral ischemia in humans [30]. The latter was recently confirmed by the Cooperative Studies on Brain Injury Depolarizations (COSBID) [31]. SD is characterized by a massive depolarization of all types of nerve cells and spreads through the cortex by contiguity with the surrounding brain tissue and is the pathophysiological component of EBI in SAH [32, 33]. SD is present in several diseases, such as migraine with aura, subdural hematoma, intraparenchymal hemorrhage, traumatic brain injury (TBI) and SAH, with a wide spectrum of clinical symptoms, which may or may not generate secondary brain injury, due to the influx of intracellular water and cytotoxic edema [32].

Studies in animal models show that SD is triggered when a sufficiently strong stimulus simultaneously depolarizes a critical minimum volume of brain tissue. The depolarizing stimulus overloads extracellular K^+ clearance mechanisms, causing extracellular K^+ to exceed a critical threshold concentration. These thresholds may vary in different species and brain regions, depending on neuronal and excitatory synaptic density, age and other factors. The inciting event causes a sudden drop in membrane resistance through the opening of ion channels. As a result, intracellular and extracellular ions move along their transmembrane concentration gradients. The massive efflux of K^+ increases the extracellular concentration. To ensure transmembrane ionic balance, excess K^+ is reciprocated by cellular influx of Na^+ and Cl^- which pulls water, causing cell swelling [32]. Depolarization also triggers Ca^{2+} influx and a more than 10-fold drop in extracellular concentration, which, along with Na^+ and water influx, leads to the release of many neurotransmitters and neuromodulators within depolarized tissue. Extracellular concentrations of glutamate, aspartate, glycine, gamma-aminobutyric acid (GABA) and taurine increase during SD. The massive increase of these substances is capable of depolarizing neighboring cells and is the critical factor for the contiguous propagation of the depolarizing wave [33]. Elevated extracellular levels of glutamate, a strongly depolarizing excitatory amino acid, further fuel DS and facilitate its propagation by activating N-methyl D-aspartate (NMDA) receptors [34, 35]. In healthy brain tissue, this ionic redistribution is self-limiting. A number of mechanisms, including Na^+ -K^+-ATPase, intracellular Ca^{2+} buffering and vascular clearance, help restore homeostasis within minutes. In humans without acute injury, the brain hemodynamic response results only in cerebral hyperemia. However, since these processes are highly dependent on glucose and oxygen, that is, high cerebral metabolic rate [35], in the scenario of acute brain injury, as in SAH, areas that are more susceptible evolve with greater tissue damage and ischemia [36].

The gold standard for SD detection is intracranial electrocorticography (ECoG), with records captured through implanted subdural electrodes [37]. The development of less invasive methods would help expand the number of centers capable of detecting SD. When intracranial ECoG is recorded simultaneously with scalp electroencephalogram (EEG), correlations were found between the two modalities. However, it has not yet been possible to detect SDs with good enough reliability with scalp EEG alone [37].

There is a high association between SD, tissue damage and functional outcomes in SAH. Currently, one of the most discussed therapies has been the use of the NMDA receptor antagonist ketamine [38]. Small retrospective studies support its use in SAH, however, there are no randomized clinical trials that provide robust evidence of its benefit. An interesting retrospective cohort study of 66 SAH patients strongly suggests that its use is beneficial. Thirty-three of 66 patients received ketamine during electrocorticographic neuromonitoring of SD in neurointensive therapy. The decision to administer ketamine depended on the need for deeper sedation, therefore, patients receiving ketamine were expected to have a worse clinical outcome. However, in patients who received ketamine, a significant decrease in the incidence of SD was seen when the infusion was started ($p < 0.001$). Even if functional outcomes are not evaluated, such work provides the basis for the production of a randomized multicenter study for this intervention [39].

Another promising therapeutic option is the PDE-III inhibitor cilostazol. The proposed mechanism of this medication is to reduce SD, due to better neurovascular coupling and improved cerebral blood flow (CBF). A randomized trial involving 50 patients with SAH on ECoG monitoring found a significant reduction in SD with cilostazol [40]. Such a study also provides support for larger studies.

2.3 Neuroinflammation

Neuroinflammation plays an important role in cell damage after aneurysmal rupture. Several inflammatory mediators, for example, interleukin-1β (IL-1β),

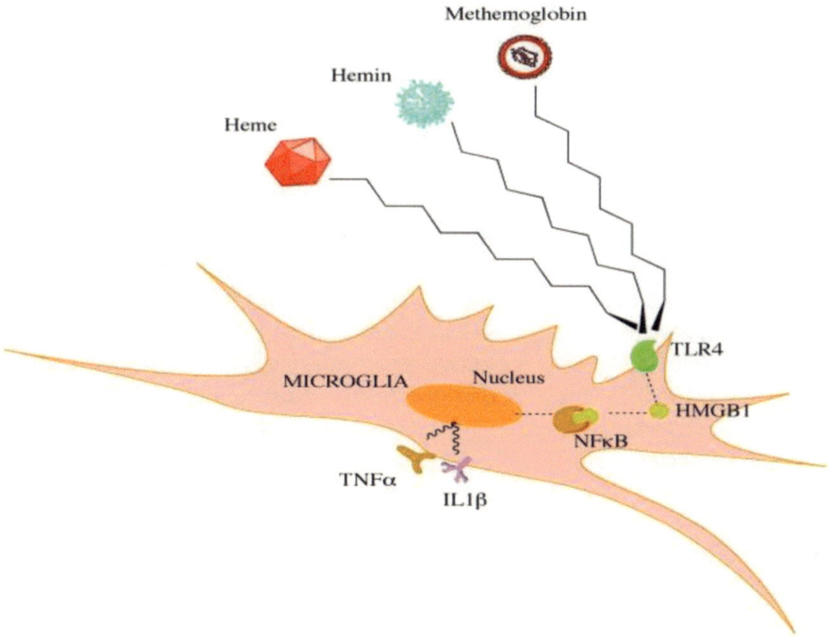

Figure 2.
The breakdown of red blood cells causes the release of heme, hemin and methemoglobin. Through interactions with TRL4 in microglia, HMGB1 is increased. This increase leads to downstream activation of NF-κB and the release of pro-inflammatory cytokines. Reprinted from Luck-Wold et al., International Journal of Molecular Sciences, 2016 [41].

interleukin-6 (IL-6) and tumor necrosis factor α (TNFα) are released in both serum and CSF in the first hours after SAH. The products of erythrocyte degradation in the subarachnoid space lead to the accumulation of hemoglobin and its products, which activate the toll-like receptor 4 (TLR4), initiating the inflammatory cascade (**Figure 2**) [41]. At that moment, one of the most important immune cells of the central nervous system (CNS) is activated: the microglia. They play a fundamental role in the pathophysiological process of EBI, as precursors of neuroinflammation. Activated microglia promote the process of endothelial adhesion, recruiting inflammatory cells to the subarachnoid space (neutrophils and macrophages), leading to BBB injury, apoptosis and neuronal edema, in addition to the production of inflammatory cytokines [42]. In SAH, TLR4 expressed by microglia is activated by ligands such as high-mobility group box protein 1 (HMGB1), heme and methemoglobin and mediates a series of intracellular pathways involving nuclear factor-κB (NF-κB) activation. After stimulation by these molecules, microglia initiate the production of pro-inflammatory cytokines, such as TNF-α, interleukins IL-1β, IL-6, interleukin-8 (IL-8) and interleukin-12 (IL-12), that result in tissue necrosis [43].

IL-1, in particular, increases BBB permeability, glial-mediated neurotoxicity and promotes ischemic changes after SAH in preclinical models [44]. IL-6, on the other hand, has a strong correlation with worse outcomes in SAH. One study was able to correlate elevated serum levels of IL-6 with measures of baseline parameters of brain injury, that is, cerebral edema scores based on imaging studies (Computerized Tomography) and the patient's respective Hunt and Hess grade [45]. In another study, there was also a correlation between higher serum levels of IL-6 in the CSF in cases with grade 4 bleeding vs. 3 by Fisher and in patients with World Federation of

Neurological Societies (WFNS) grade 5 SAH, suggesting that the role of IL-6 signaling in the early inflammatory response is a sensitive biomarker of early brain injury. In addition, high levels of IL-6 for more than 72 hours after the injury are correlated with worse outcomes [11]. Published in 2015, an interesting study based on neuromonitoring with cerebral microdialysis identified higher concentrations of IL-6 in the brain compared to systemic concentrations, corroborating the hypothesis of cerebral compartmentalization. In it, there was still an association of high levels of IL-6 with GCS, metabolic disorder and cerebral perfusion pressure (CPP) lower than 70 mmhg [46].

Other substances involved in the neuroinflammation process are matrix metalloproteinases (MMPs), especially MMP-9. The loss of BBB integrity is related to the upregulation of these proteinases in aHSA and is related to the pathophysiology of EBI [41]. In animal models with rats, increased expression was associated with apoptosis of hippocampal neurons [47]. Increased expression and subsequent activation of MMP-9 may occur in response to reactive oxygen species and pro-inflammatory cytokines such as TNF-a and interleukin-17 (IL-17). The source of MMP-9 in SAH is not well described, but evidence obtained from ischemia-reperfusion models indicates that neutrophils may be the main source of MMP-9 acting on the BBB [48]. MMP-9 can also drive neuroinflammation through activation of pro-inflammatory signals and clotting factors, triggering a positive feedback loop that promotes thromboinflammation and neurotoxicity [49]. The increase of MMP-9 in the CSF by cerebral microdialysis techniques correlates with the extent of EBI, vasospasm and DCI [46].

Faced with this pathophysiological hypothesis, drugs with cerebral anti-inflammatory action were studied to improve the outcome of SAH in the acute phase. A study carried out at the University of Zurich, involving 138 patients, showed that the use of non-steroidal anti-inflammatory drugs (NSAIDs) (acetaminophen, dipyrone, diclofenac and ibuprofen) independently reduced serum levels of IL-6 and CRP, as well as obtained better functional outcomes [50]. Another drug studied in this context was heparin. Despite its anticoagulant effect, this polysaccharide from the glycosaminoglycan family has a pleiotropic effect, showing broad anti-inflammatory

Medication	Mechanism	Potential benefit
Clazosentan	Selective antagonist of Endothelin receptors	Vasospasm reduction
Nitric oxide (NO)	Relaxation of endothelial smooth muscle cells via cGMP	Vasodilation
Sildenafil	PDE-V inhibitor	Vasodilation
Cilostazol	PDE-III inhibitor	Neurovascular coupling
Milrinone	PDE-III inhibitor	Vasodilation
Magnesium Sulfate	Blocks intracellular calcium influx and improves blood rheological function	Vasodilation, neuroprotection and increased cerebral blood flow
Ketamine	Blocking NMDA receptors	Reduction of propagation of excitatory stimuli
NSAIDs	Reduction of circulating levels of IL 6 and CRP	Decreased brain inflammatory response
Heparin	Anti-inflammatory and immunomodulatory activity	Decreased brain inflammatory response

Table 1.
Summarizes the main study medications and potential beneficial effects in the treatment of EBI.

and immunomodulatory activity, even at doses that do not cause anticoagulation. An animal study showed that low-dose heparin is able to attenuate neuroinflammation in SAH [51]. **Table 1** summarizes the main drugs studied for the treatment of EBI.

3. Conclusion

The pathophysiological knowledge of SAH is of fundamental importance to promote paradigm shifts and new therapeutic proposals for this devastating disease. In the last 20 years, the paradigm that ischemic lesions secondary to aneurysmal rupture started only after the third day fell apart with the emergence of the new concept of EBI. A pathology with enormous morbidity and mortality for years, with great financial and social impact, requires new therapeutic weapons. Clazosentan, ketamine, cilostazol, non-steroidal anti-inflammatory drugs and heparin have shown to be possible options, but they require larger studies to consolidate their applications.

Acknowledgements

I thank everyone who participated in this work, especially my wife, MD Karylla Marques for her unconditional support and Dr. Salomón Rojas, my master and great friend, for teaching me to walk in the paths of neurointensivism.

Conflicts of interest

The authors declare that there are no conflicts of interest of any kind.

Acronyms

ATP	adenosine triphosphate
BBB	blood-brain barrier
CBF	cerebral blood flow
cGMP	cyclic guanosine monophosphate
CNS	central nervous system
CPP	cerebral perfusion pressure
CPR	C-reactive protein
CSF	Cerebrospinal fluid
DCI	delayed cerebral ischemia
EBI	early brain injury
ECoG	electrocorticography
EEG	electroencephalogram
eNOS	endothelial NOS
ET 1	endothelin-1
GABA	gamma-aminobutyric acid
GCS	Glasgow coma scale
HMGB1	high-mobility group box protein 1
ICP	intracranial pressure
IL-1 β	interleukin-1β

IL-12	interleukin-12
IL-17	interleukin-17
IL-6	interleukin-6
IL-8	interleukin-8
iNOS	inducible NOS
MCA	middle cerebral artery
MMP-9	metalloproteinases-9
MMPs	metalloproteinases
NF-κB	nuclear factor-κB
NIHSS	National institutes of health stroke scale
NMDA	N-methyl D-aspartate
nNOS	neural NOS
NO	Nitric oxide
NOS	Nitric oxide synthase
NSAIDs	non-steroidal anti-inflammatory drugs
PDE-III	phosphodiesterase III
PDE-V	phosphodiesterase V
SAH	subarachnoid hemorrhage
SD	spreading depolarizations
TBI	traumatic brain injury
TEG	thromboelastography
TNFα	tumor necrosis factor α
TRL4	toll-like receptor 4
WFNS	world federation of neurological societies

Author details

Guilherme Nascimento de Morais* and Salomón Rojas
Hospital Beneficência Portuguesa de São Paulo, São Paulo, Brazil

*Address all correspondence to: nascimento.guilherme@hotmail.com

References

[1] Rincon F, Rossenwasser RH, Dumont A. The epidemiology of admissions of nontraumatic subarachnoid hemorrhage in the United States. Neurosurgery 2013; 73(2):217-22; discussion 212-3. DOI: 10.1227/01.neu.0000430290.93304.33

[2] Suarez JI, Tarr RW, Selman WR. Aneurysmal subarachnoid hemorrhage. The New England Journal of Medicine. 2006;**354**(4):387-396. DOI: 10.1056/NEJMra052732

[3] Kusaka G, Ishikawa M, Nanda A, Granger DN, Zhang JH. Signaling pathways for early brain injury after subarachnoid hemorrhage. Journal of Cerebral Blood Flow and Metabolism. 2004;**24**(8):916-925. DOI: 10.1097/01.WCB.0000125886.48838.7E

[4] Rapoport RM. Bilirubin oxidation products and cerebral vasoconstriction. Frontiers in Pharmacology. 2018;**9**:303. DOI: 10.3389/fphar.2018.00303

[5] Vergouwen MD, Vermeulen M, van Gijn J, Rinkel GJ, Wijdicks EF, Muizelaar JP, et al. Definition of delayed cerebral ischemia after aneurysmal subarachnoid hemorrhage as an outcome event in clinical trials and observational studies: Proposal of a multidisciplinary research group. Stroke. 2010;**41**(10):2391-2395. DOI: 10.1161/STROKEAHA.110.589275

[6] Macdonald RL. Delayed neurological deterioration after subarachnoid haemorrhage. Nature Reviews. Neurology. 2014;**10**(1):44-58. DOI: 10.1038/nrneurol.2013.246. Epub 2013 Dec 10

[7] Davenport AP, Hyndman KA, Dhaun N, Southan C, Kohan DE, Pollock JS, et al. Endothelin. Pharmacological Reviews. 2016;**68**(2):357-418. DOI: 10.1124/pr.115.011833

[8] Macdonald RL, Kassell NF, Mayer S, Ruefenacht D, Schmiedek P, Weidauer S, et al. CONSCIOUS-1 investigators. Clazosentan to overcome neurological ischemia and infarction occurring after subarachnoid hemorrhage (CONSCIOUS-1): Randomized, double-blind, placebo-controlled phase 2 dose-finding trial. Stroke. 2008;**39**(11):3015-3021. DOI: 10.1161/STROKEAHA.108.519942. Epub 2008 Aug 7

[9] Macdonald RL, Higashida RT, Keller E, Mayer SA, Molyneux A, Raabe A, et al. Clazosentan, an endothelin receptor antagonist, in patients with aneurysmal subarachnoid haemorrhage and surgical clipping: A randomized, double-blind, placebo-controlled phase 3 trial (CONSCIOUS-2). Lancet Neurology. 2011;**10**(7):618-625. DOI: 10.1016/S1474-4422(11)70108-9. Epub 2011 Jun 2

[10] Geraghty JR, Davis JL, Testai FD. Neuroinflammation and microvascular dysfunction after experimental subarachnoid hemorrhage: Emerging components of early brain injury related to outcome. Neurocritical Care. 2019;**31**(2):373-389. DOI: 10.1007/s12028-019-00710-x

[11] Rass V, Helbok R. Early brain injury after poor-grade subarachnoid hemorrhage. Current Neurology and Neuroscience Reports. 2019;**19**(10):78. DOI: 10.1007/s11910-019-0990-3

[12] Przykaza Ł. Understanding the connection between common stroke comorbidities, their associated inflammation, and the course of

the cerebral ischemia/reperfusion cascade. Frontiers in Immunology. 2021;**12**:782569. DOI: 10.3389/fimmu.2021.782569

[13] Dienel A, Kumar TP, Blackburn SL, McBride DW. Role of platelets in the pathogenesis of delayed injury after subarachnoid hemorrhage. Journal of Cerebral Blood Flow and Metabolism. 2021;**41**(11):2820-2830. DOI: 10.1177/0271678X211020865. Epub 2021 Jun 10

[14] Hijdra A, Van Gijn J, Stefanko S, Van Dongen KJ, Vermeulen M, Van Crevel H. Delayed cerebral ischemia after aneurysmal subarachnoid hemorrhage: Clinicoanatomical correlations. Neurology. 1986;**36**(3):329-333. DOI: 10.1212/wnl.36.3.329

[15] Wellman GC, Koide M. Impact of subarachnoid hemorrhage on parenchymal arteriolar function. Acta Neurochirurgica. Supplement. 2013;**115**:173-177. DOI: 10.1007/978-3-7091-1192-5_33

[16] Xu HL, Garcia M, Testai F, Vetri F, Barabanova A, Pelligrino DA, et al. Pharmacologic blockade of vascular adhesion protein-1 lessens neurologic dysfunction in rats subjected to subarachnoid hemorrhage. Brain Research. 2014;**1586**:83-89. DOI: 10.1016/j.brainres.2014.08.036. Epub 2014 Aug 29

[17] Friedrich B, Müller F, Feiler S, Schöller K, Plesnila N. Experimental subarachnoid hemorrhage causes early and long-lasting microarterial constriction and microthrombosis: An in-vivo microscopy study. Journal of Cerebral Blood Flow and Metabolism. 2012;**32**(3):447-455. DOI: 10.1038/jcbfm.2011.154. Epub 2011 Dec 7

[18] Sabri M, AiJ LK, Macdonald RL. Mechanisms of microthrombosis and microcirculatory constriction after experimental subarachnoid hemorrhage. Acta Neurochirurgica. Supplement. 2013;**115**:185-192. DOI: 10.1007/978-3-7091-1192-5_35

[19] Friedrich V, Flores R, Muller A, Sehba FA. Luminal platelet aggregates in functional deficits in parenchymal vessels after subarachnoid hemorrhage. Brain Research. 2010;**1354**:179-187. DOI: 10.1016/j.brainres.2010.07.040. Epub 2010 Jul 21

[20] Frontera JA, Provencio JJ, Sehba FA, McIntyre TM, Nowacki AS, Gordon E, et al. The role of platelet activation and inflammation in early brain injury following subarachnoid hemorrhage. Neurocritical Care. 2017;**26**(1):48-57. DOI: 10.1007/s12028-016-0292-4

[21] Iqbal S, Hayman EG, Hong C, Stokum JA, Kurland DB, Gerzanich V, et al. Inducible nitric oxide synthase (NOS-2) in subarachnoid hemorrhage: Regulatory mechanisms and therapeutic implications. Brain Circ. 2016;**2**(1):8-19. DOI: 10.4103/2394-8108.178541

[22] Bruder N, Higashida R, Santin-Janin H, Dubois C, Aldrich EF, Marr A, et al. The REACT study: Design of a randomized phase 3 trial to assess the efficacy and safety of clazosentan for preventing deterioration due to delayed cerebral ischemia after aneurysmal subarachnoid hemorrhage. BMC Neurology. 2022;**22**(1):492. DOI: 10.1186/s12883-022-03002-8

[23] Lee A. Clazosentan: First approval. Drugs. 2022;**82**(6):697-702. DOI: 10.1007/s40265-022-01708-0

[24] Sehba FA, Friedrich V. Cerebral microvasculature is an early target of subarachnoid hemorrhage. Acta Neurochirurgica. Supplement. 2013;**115**:199-205. DOI: 10.1007/978-3-7091-1192-5_37

[25] Cerqueira NF, Yoshida WB. Nitric oxide: Review. Acta Cirúrgica Brasileira. 2022;**2022**(6):17. DOI: 10.1590/S0102-86502002000600011

[26] Terpolilli NA, Feiler S, Dienel A, Müller F, Heumos N, Friedrich B, et al. Nitric oxide inhalation reduces brain damage, prevents mortality, and improves neurological outcome after subarachnoid hemorrhage by resolving early pial microvasospasms. Journal of Cerebral Blood Flow and Metabolism. 2016;**36**(12):2096-2107. DOI: 10.1177/0271678X15605848. Epub 2015 Nov 2

[27] Washington CW, Derdeyn CP, Dhar R, Arias EJ, Chicoine MR, Cross DT, et al. A phase I proof-of-concept and safety trial of sildenafil to treat cerebral vasospasm following subarachnoid hemorrhage. Journal of Neurosurgery. 2016;**124**(2): 318-327. DOI: 10.3171/2015.2.JNS142752. Epub 2015 Aug 28

[28] Lakhal K, Hivert A, Alexandre PL, Fresco M, Robert-Edan V, Rodie-Talbere PA, et al. Intravenous milrinone for cerebral vasospasm in subarachnoid hemorrhage: The MILRISPASM controlled before-after study. Neurocritical Care. 2021;**35**(3):669-679. DOI: 10.1007/s12028-021-01331-z. Epub 2021 Sep 3

[29] Kunze E, Lilla N, Stetter C, Ernestus RI, Westermaier T. Magnesium protects in episodes of critical perfusion after aneurysmal SAH. Translational Neuroscience. 2018;**9**:99-105. DOI: 10.1515/tnsci-2018-0016

[30] Leo AA. Spreading depression of activity in the cerebral cortex. Journal of Neurophysiology. 1944;7(6):359-390

[31] Dohmen C, Sakowitz OW, Fabricius M, Bosche B, Reithmeier T, Ernestus RI, et al. Spreading depolarizations occur in human ischemic stroke with high incidence. Annals of Neurology: Official Journal of the American Neurological Association and the Child Neurology Society. 2008;**63**(6):720-728

[32] Ayata C, Lauritzen M. Spreading depression, spreading depolarizations, and the cerebral vasculature. Physiological Reviews. 2015;**95**(3):953-993. DOI: 10.1152/physrev.00027.2014

[33] Eriksen N, Rostrup E, Fabricius M, Scheel M, Major S, Winkler MKL, et al. Early focal brain injury after subarachnoid hemorrhage correlates with spreading depolarizations. Neurology. 2019;**92**(4):e326-e341. DOI: 10.1212/WNL.0000000000006814. Epub 2018 Dec 28

[34] Molchanova S, Kööbi P, Oja SS, Saransaari P. Interstitial concentrations of amino acids in the rat striatum during global forebrain ischemia and potassium-evoked spreading depression. Neurochemical Research. 2004;**29**(8):1519-1527. DOI: 10.1023/b:nere.0000029564.98905.5c

[35] Sakowitz OW, Santos E, Nagel A, Krajewski KL, Hertle DN, Vajkoczy P, et al. Clusters of spreading depolarizations are associated with disturbed cerebral metabolism in patients with aneurysmal subarachnoid hemorrhage. Stroke. 2013;**44**(1):220-223. DOI: 10.1161/STROKEAHA.112.672352. Epub 2012 Dec 6

[36] Dreier JP. The role of spreading depression, spreading depolarization and spreading ischemia in neurological disease. Nature Medicine. 2011;**17**(4):439-447. DOI: 10.1038/nm.2333. Epub 2011 Apr 7

[37] Hartings JA, Li C, Hinzman JM, Shuttleworth CW, Ernst GL, Dreier JP, et al. Direct current electrocorticography

for clinical neuromonitoring of spreading depolarizations. Journal of Cerebral Blood Flow and Metabolism. 2017;**37**(5):1857-1870. DOI: 10.1177/0271678X16653135. Epub 2016 Jan 1

[38] Hertle DN, Dreier JP, Woitzik J, Hartings JA, Bullock R, Okonkwo DO, et al. Cooperative study of brain injury depolarizations (COSBID). Effect of analgesics and sedatives on the occurrence of spreading depolarizations with acute brain injury. Brain. 2012;**135**(Pt 8):2390-2398. DOI: 10.1093/brain/aws152. Epub 2012 Jun 19

[39] Santos E, Olivares-Rivera A, Major S, Sánchez-Porras R, Uhlmann L, Kunzmann K, et al. Lasting s-ketamine block of spreading depolarizations in subarachnoid hemorrhage: A retrospective cohort study. Critical Care. 2019;**23**(1):427. DOI: 10.1186/s13054-019-2711-3

[40] Sugimoto K, Nomura S, Shirao S, Inoue T, Ishihara H, Kawano R, et al. Cilostazol decreases duration of spreading depolarization and spreading ischemia after aneurysmal subarachnoid hemorrhage. Annals of Neurology. 2018;**84**(6):873-885. DOI: 10.1002/ana.25361. Epub 2018 Nov 29

[41] Lucke-Wold BP, Logsdon AF, Manoranjan B, Turner RC, McConnell E, Vates GE, et al. Aneurysmal subarachnoid hemorrhage and neuroinflammation: A comprehensive review. International Journal of Molecular Sciences. 2016;**17**(4):497. DOI: 10.3390/ijms17040497

[42] Wang XY, Wu F, Zhan RY, Zhou HJ. Inflammatory role of microglia in brain injury caused by subarachnoid hemorrhage. Frontiers in Cellular Neuroscience. 2022;**16**:956185. DOI: 10.3389/fncel.2022.956185

[43] Kawakita F, Fujimoto M, Liu L, Nakano F, Nakatsuka Y, Suzuki H. Effects of toll-like receptor 4 antagonists against cerebral vasospasm after experimental subarachnoid hemorrhage in mice. Molecular Neurobiology. 2017;**54**(8):6624-6633. DOI: 10.1007/s12035-016-0178-7. Epub 2016 Oct 13

[44] Thornton P, Pinteaux E, Gibson RM, Allan SM, Rothwell NJ. Interleukin-1-induced neurotoxicity is mediated by glia and requires caspase activation and free radical release. Journal of Neurochemistry. 2006;**98**(1):258-266. DOI: 10.1111/j.1471-4159.2006.03872.x

[45] Savarraj J, Parsha K, Hergenroeder G, Ahn S, Chang TR, Kim DH, et al. Early brain injury associated with systemic inflammation after subarachnoid hemorrhage. Neurocritical Care. 2018;**28**(2):203-211. DOI: 10.1007/s12028-017-0471-y

[46] Helbok R, Schiefecker AJ, Beer R, Dietmann A, Antunes AP, Sohm F, et al. Early brain injury after aneurysmal subarachnoid hemorrhage: A multimodal neuromonitoring study. Critical Care. 2015;**19**(1):75. DOI: 10.1186/s13054-015-0809-9

[47] Guo Z, Sun X, He Z, Jiang Y, Zhang X. Role of matrix metalloproteinase-9 in apoptosis of hippocampal neurons in rats during early brain injury after subarachnoid hemorrhage. Neurological Sciences. 2010;**31**(2):143-149. DOI: 10.1007/s10072-009-0192-x. Epub 2009 Dec 24

[48] Hayman EG, Wessell A, Gerzanich V, Sheth KN, Simard JM. Mechanisms of global cerebral edema formation in aneurysmal subarachnoid hemorrhage. Neurocritical Care. 2017;**26**(2):301-310. DOI: 10.1007/s12028-016-0354-7

[49] Rempe RG, Hartz AMS, Bauer B. Matrix metalloproteinases

in the brain and blood-brain barrier: Versatile breakers and makers. Journal of Cerebral Blood Flow and Metabolism. 2016;**36**(9):1481-1507. DOI: 10.1177/0271678X16655551. Epub 2016 Jun 20

[50] Muroi C, Hugelshofer M, Seule M, Keller E. The impact of nonsteroidal anti-inflammatory drugs on inflammatory response after aneurysmal subarachnoid hemorrhage. Neurocritical Care. 2014;**20**(2):240-246. DOI: 10.1007/s12028-013-9930-2

[51] Simard JM, Tosun C, Ivanova S, Kurland DB, Hong C, Radecki L, et al. Heparin reduces neuroinflammation and transsynaptic neuronal apoptosis in a model of subarachnoid hemorrhage. Translational Stroke Research. 2012;**3**(Suppl. 1):155-165. DOI: 10.1007/s12975-012-0166-9. Epub 2012 Apr 14

Chapter 3

The Use of Artificial Intelligence in the Management of Intracranial Aneurysms

Luis Antonio Marín-Castañeda, Fernanda de Leon-Mendoza and Hector Eduardo Valdez-Ruvalcaba

Abstract

The use of artificial intelligence (AI) has potential benefits in the management of intracranial aneurysms. Early detection of intracranial aneurysms is critical due to their high risk of complications such as rupture, vasospasm, and ischemia with highly impact on morbidity and mortality. The main findings suggest that AI can improve the accuracy of aneurysm detection, rupture risk prediction, and assist neurointervention in planning and performing procedures. This chapter discusses the potential for AI to improve patient care by enabling earlier diagnosis and timely treatment, reducing medical errors, costs, morbidity, and mortality. However, further validation of AI-based applications is necessary in a real-world clinical setting.

Keywords: intracranial aneurysm, artificial intelligence, machine learning, rupture risk assessment, computer-assisted diagnosis

1. Introduction

The detection and management of unruptured intracranial aneurysms (IAs) is a significant public health concern, affecting an estimated 3–7% of the population [1, 2]. Advances in neuroimaging, such as magnetic resonance angiography (MRA), computed tomographic angiography (CTA), and digital subtraction angiography (DSA), have increased the detection of incidental aneurysms [3, 4]. However, physicians' manual measurements of aneurysm morphology on 2D/3D projections have limitations of subjectivity and inconsistency, leading to interobserver variations [1].

To enhance aneurysm management, it is crucial to strive for greater accuracy and efficacy throughout all stages. Researchers have dedicated significant effort toward identifying risk factors and developing prediction models related to aneurysm initiation, growth, rupture, and intervention assessment [1, 5]. Several scoring systems have been developed and validated, such as PHASES [6] for predicting rupture risk and ELAPSS [7] for predicting growth risk. Additionally, the UIATS [6] score has been developed to balance risks and benefits directly. However, these scoring systems focus mainly on predicting rupture events rather than providing a comprehensive range of objective predictive analytics that may be useful for shared decision-making.

The concept of artificial intelligence (AI) was first introduced by J. McCarthy in the 1950s and involves the development of algorithms that can replicate human cognitive functions, including problem-solving, reasoning, and learning [7]. In essence, it is the ability of a machine to imitate intelligent human behavior and solve complex tasks using a single algorithm or brain [8]. AI includes various subsets, such as computer vision, image processing, artificial neural networks (ANN), convolutional neural networks (CNN), machine learning (ML), and deep learning (DL) [9].

In recent years, AI has become increasingly popular in the medical field, with applications in screening, diagnosis, and risk analysis across various specialties. In the field of neuroscience, AI is used for diverse purposes, such as clinical prediction modeling in intramedullary spinal tumor surgery [10], as well as in the study of neuro-oncology [11], epilepsy [12], Alzheimer's disease [13, 14], schizophrenia [14], and other neurological disorders [15].

AI can identify potential diagnoses, select appropriate treatments based on medical records and imaging data, and make independent decisions based on training data. This technology, which relies on past experiences, has shown promising results in improving patient care by enabling earlier diagnosis and timely treatment, reducing medical errors, costs, morbidity, and mortality [16, 17]. In the 2000s, AI was introduced into the management of intracranial aneurysms, providing an automated morphological 3-D characterization as an alternative to assess the risk of rupture and to determine the most appropriate management without delay [18]. Subsequently, the implementation of artificial intelligence methods allowed for automated morphological calculation, rupture risk stratification, and outcome prediction in aneurysm assessment, demonstrating excellent performance (**Figure 1**) [7].

The goal of using AI in intracranial aneurysm management is to enhance and improve patient health care. However, not all AI studies have been validated in a real clinical setting. In a recent study by Alwalid et al. [5], the clinical feasibility of the most popular AI applications in intracranial aneurysms was evaluated. The study

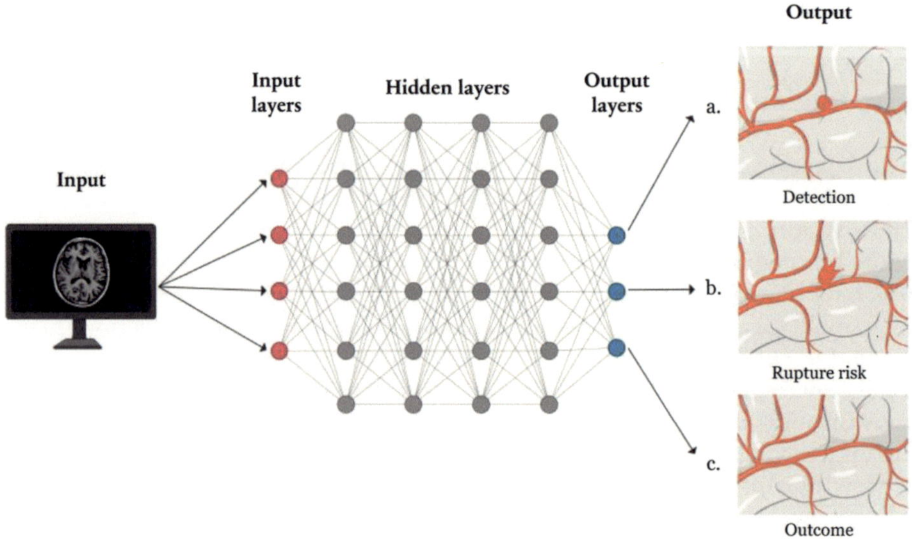

Figure 1.
Schematic representation of the use of DL-based algorithms in intracranial aneurysm management. The main applications include a. detection of intracranial aneurysms, b. assessing the risk of rupture, and c. predicting prognosis and risk of recurrence.

demonstrated that AI-based applications, particularly aneurysm detection, can potentially improve radiologists' clinical performance and shorten interpretation time. However, further validation is necessary in a real-world clinical setting [1, 5].

This chapter will discuss AI's main applications in managing intracranial aneurysms and its limitations and potential for future development.

2. Intracranial aneurysm detection

Artificial intelligence has become a significant focus in neurology for the detection of intracranial aneurysms. Early detection of aneurysms is critical due to their high risk of rupture, morbidity, and mortality. Computer-assisted diagnosis (CAD) is an AI-based technology that has emerged as a valuable tool for aneurysm detection based on imaging features. There are two types of CAD algorithms: conventional-style and deep learning-based models [19].

CAD systems have proven to be useful tools for faster, more accurate, objective, and consistent diagnoses of intracranial aneurysms by reducing intra and interobserver variability. Conventional-style CAD systems utilize quantitative analysis of predetermined imaging characteristics to detect aneurysms automatically [10]. The first CAD system developed for aneurysms using this method was created by Arimura et al. [20], which showed high sensitivity but could not detect small or fusiform aneurysms. Additionally, digital subtraction angiography (DSA) as an outside reference standard did not verify the aneurysms in the study.

Yang et al. [21] developed a fully automated algorithm for aneurysm detection that overcomes some of the limitations of conventional-style CAD systems. Their algorithm utilizes two complementary techniques: automatic intracranial artery segmentation and detecting points of interest from the segmented vessels, verified by DSA. This system demonstrated high sensitivity, especially for small aneurysms, and outperformed human detection in some cases. However, conventional-style CAD systems have a high false positive rate and low sensitivity, which limits their reliability and widespread adoption in clinical practice [19].

DL-based models for intracranial aneurysm detection have shown significant improvements in sensitivity and specificity compared to conventional-style CAD systems. These models can detect aneurysms of various shapes and sizes and can differentiate them from normal vessels and other intracranial structures with high accuracy. Furthermore, DL-based CAD systems can segment and quantify aneurysms, providing valuable information for treatment planning. DL models for aneurysm detection can be trained on a large dataset of radiological images, allowing for the identification of subtle imaging features that may be missed by human observers. For example, DL models can identify aneurysms in regions of the brain that are difficult to visualize or differentiate small aneurysms from normal vasculature [22, 23].

DL-based CAD systems have shown promising results in intracranial aneurysm detection. In 2018, Hua et al. developed a DL-based system that achieved a sensitivity of 96.4% and a specificity of 91.1% for aneurysm detection on MRA images. In another study, Zhang et al. developed a DL-based system that achieved a sensitivity of 92.3% and a specificity of 95.2% for aneurysm detection on CTA images [24]. These DL-based CAD systems have the potential to improve the accuracy and efficiency of aneurysm detection greatly. These models can be classified according to whether they have been developed for MRA, CTA, or DSA. REF.

2.1 MRA-based models

In recent years, several DL-based computer-assisted diagnosis (CAD) algorithms that use deep learning and magnetic resonance angiography (MRA) have emerged. One such algorithm, called DeepMedic, was developed by Sichtermann et al. [25] for automated detection of intracranial aneurysms using 3D time-of-flight MRA. The algorithm achieved a sensitivity rate of 90%, with higher sensitivity rates of 96% and 100% for aneurysms measuring between 3 and 7 mm and >7 mm, respectively. However, the algorithm showed poor specificity due to the limited sample size. The study also compared the performance of two clinicians in detecting aneurysms with and without augmentation from the DeepMedic algorithm, revealing improved sensitivity when the human reader was combined with the algorithm [19, 25].

Stember et al. [26] machined a convolutional neural network (CNN) algorithm for detecting intracranial aneurysms (IA) on both time-of-flight MRA and contrast-enhanced MRA. Their algorithm achieved a high sensitivity rate of 98.8%, but during the learning process, it only incorporated two-dimensional maximum intensity projection (MIP) images, resulting in false positives due to vascular curvatures that mimic aneurysms. In another study, Ueda et al. [27] developed an 18-layer CNN algorithm that utilized imaging data from multiple MRI units from various institutions. The algorithm achieved a sensitivity rate of 91–93% for aneurysms that are smaller than 5 mm. However, due to the heterogeneous internal signals of large aneurysms that are greater than 5 mm, the sensitivity rate was not satisfactory for this type of aneurysm [28]. Algorithms that use deep learning and magnetic resonance angiography (MRA) have shown promising results for the automated detection of intracranial aneurysms.

2.2 CTA-based models

Compared to MRA-based models, fewer studies have proposed AI algorithms for detecting intracranial aneurysms on CT angiography. In 2019, Park and colleagues introduced a DL-based CAD system called HeadXNet, which was applied to CTA images and outperformed clinicians in aneurysm detection [29]. Another study by Yang et al. [30] proposed an 18-layer CNN DL algorithm on CTA, which had a high sensitivity of 97.5% but a high false positive rate. Nevertheless, this algorithm helped improve the detection rate of IAs smaller than 3 mm, which are often missed by humans.

The DeepMedic algorithm developed by Sichtermann and colleagues in 2019 has also been applied to CTA images for aneurysmal subarachnoid hemorrhage, with a sensitivity of 87% and false positives of 0.42 for aneurysms larger than 30 mm and a sensitivity of 96% and a false positive of 0.14 for aneurysms larger than 100 mm [19].

2.3 DSA-based models

Several AI models have been developed to automatically detect intracranial aneurysms on 2D and 3D-DSA. In 2020, Jin and colleagues [31] developed a U-shaped deep neural network for aneurysmal detection and segmentation on 2D-DSA, which showed a high lesion-level sensitivity and low false-positive rate, making it a useful clinical tool for prompt diagnosis with less risk of errors. Duan and colleagues in 2019 [32] developed the regional average grayscale suppression (RAGS) algorithm for dual-input 2D DSA images, achieving a sensitivity of 100%, but with 11 false positives per case. However, combining dual-input images with the RAGS algorithm reduced false positives to 1.8 per case [19].

In summary, computer-aided detection of intracranial aneurysms using deep learning and medical imaging techniques has shown promising results for improving diagnostic accuracy and reducing false negatives. MRA-based models have been extensively studied and have demonstrated high sensitivity rates but poor specificity. CTA-based models have shown comparable sensitivity rates to MRA-based models, with fewer studies reported in the literature. DSA-based models have also shown high sensitivity rates, with low false positives, but require more invasive imaging procedures [19].

However, the performance of these algorithms can be affected by various factors, such as the quality and quantity of training data, machine learning approach, and image processing techniques. Further research is necessary to optimize these algorithms and develop reliable and efficient tools for detecting and diagnosing intracranial aneurysms [5].

3. Treatment outcomes

Aneurysms can be treated using surgical or endovascular techniques. However, there is still a risk of stroke or death, ranging from 3 to 10%, even with proper treatment [33].

Size, location, and morphology must be considered to determine the best treatment for an aneurysm [5]. For aneurysms located in distal segments or at the middle cerebral artery trifurcation, surgical therapy may be preferred. On the other hand, endovascular treatment has shown better results for proximal intracranial carotid and posterior circulation aneurysms. In some cases, very large or complex aneurysms may require a combination of endovascular and surgical techniques [34].

The use of artificial intelligence (AI) has enabled the determination of the most suitable intervention therapy based on patient characteristics and aneurysm features. Through the analysis of large datasets, AI models can assist in the decision-making process. Moreover, incorporating objective data on aneurysm flow and morphological characteristics can further enhance the process, improving occlusion rates and potentially reducing the risk of recanalization [35].

3.1 Surgery

The application of artificial intelligence (AI) in neurosurgery has generated considerable interest in recent years, mainly due to the large amounts of data produced by modern diagnostic methods that require quantitative analysis. In conjunction with advancements in microsurgical techniques, the use of surgical management involving the placement of a clip across the neck of a cerebral aneurysm has proven to be an effective and safe procedure for patients with unruptured cerebral aneurysms or subarachnoid hemorrhage (SAH) [36].

Certain factors could influence prognosis, and studies have indicated that patients treated at specialized neurosurgical centers with high volumes of cerebral aneurysm procedures tend to experience better outcomes than those treated at lower-volume centers. Numerous studies have shown that machine learning (ML) can be utilized in surgical procedures, including presurgical planning, intraoperative guidance, and outcome prediction [34, 36, 37].

Staartjes and colleagues used various ML models, including support vector machines, decision trees, random forests, generalized linear models, generalized additive models, and stochastic gradient boosting machines, to achieve a peak accuracy of 91% during internal validation of the gradient boosting machine [8].

Neurosurgeons can incorporate AI and ML into their daily clinical practices and use these models for intraoperative and postoperative care, thereby creating superior medical care and research tools and techniques [38].

3.2 Endovascular therapy

The techniques used for endovascular therapy for cerebral aneurysms have evolved, with coil systems being introduced in the early 1990s [39], and newer techniques, including stent-assisted coiling, balloon-assisted coiling, flow diverters (FD), disruptors, and new embolic materials, such as liquids, showing promising results [33]. However, complications can occur, such as intraprocedural aneurysm rupture and thromboembolism, which are more frequent in the setting of SAH compared to unruptured aneurysms [40].

Flow diverters have emerged as an alternative to coil embolization for treating wide-neck and challenging aneurysm morphologies, but 25% of FD-treated intracranial aneurysms still fail to reach complete occlusion even after six months, increasing the risk of rupture and thromboembolic complications. Factors such as aneurysm ostium size, pre- and post-treatment inflow rates, shear rate, and averaged velocity are analyzed to assess the effectiveness of FD treatment [40].

For coil embolization, recanalization has been shown to correlate with aneurysm morphometrics such as size, neck-to-dome ratio, and neck size, which have been used to gauge coil treatment outcomes [41]. On the other hand, the FD treatment of IAs does not correlate to these morphological features; instead, hemodynamic metrics are analyzed [42].

Mut et al. [43] found that specific hemodynamic metrics, such as pre-and post-treatment inflow rates, shear rate, and aneurysm velocity, significantly differed between occluded and non-occluded intracranial aneurysms following six months of FD treatment.

Paliwal et al. used computational image analysis to extract information on morphology, hemodynamics, and FD-device characteristics from FD-treated aneurysms [44]. They used this data to train machine learning algorithms to predict 6-month clinical outcomes after FD treatment, finding that a neural network performed best (AUC = 0.967) and that the G-SVM with NN was able to predict occlusion outcomes with 90% accuracy.

Guedon et al. [45] utilized ElasticNet penalized logistic regression for developing a predictive score consisting of aneurysm diameter, treatment indication, parent artery diameter ratio, neck ratio, side-branch artery, and sex to forecast aneurysm occlusion following FD treatment at a follow-up of six months or longer, achieving an accuracy of 86%.

Endovascular therapy for cerebral aneurysms has undergone significant advancements over the years, with newer techniques, such as flow diverters showing promising results for treating challenging aneurysm morphologies. However, complications can still arise, and effective treatment outcome assessment requires considering various factors such as hemodynamic metrics and morphological features.

4. Prediction of aneurysm complications

The cornerstone of prediction modeling in aneurysm is to predict rupture, and statistical models such as logistic regression have been widely used for this purpose [35]. However, recent studies have demonstrated that machine learning (ML) models perform better than traditional statistical methods because they can process massive amounts of data and model nonlinear relationships [46].

Hemodynamics is considered the most valuable parameter in exploring intracranial aneurysm behavior. Promising AI tools, such as computational fluid dynamics, have been developed to assess hemodynamics [47]. Morphological features, including size and shape, have shown great potential in identifying aneurysms at risk of rupture, while geometric features that describe the 3D characteristics of the aneurysm can be automated to evaluate aneurysm formation, growth, and risk of rupture. Integrating clinical, morphological, and hemodynamic parameters can improve rupture prediction, but limited clinical use is still observed due to complexity, cost, and expertise requirements [5].

Several studies have used ML methods to predict complications arising from aneurysm rupture, such as vasospasm, delayed cerebral ischemia, and infarction [48]. Dumon et al. [49] developed an ANN prediction model that had a higher predictive value (AUC of 0.960) for symptomatic cerebral vasospasm than two multiple logistic regression models (AUC = 0.933 and 0.897). In another study, ML methods such as SVM, random forest, and multilayer perceptron outperformed logistic regression models in predicting delayed cerebral ischemia.

Tanioka et al. [47] used random forests to develop early prediction models for delayed cerebral ischemia, angiographic vasospasm, and cerebral infarction using clinical variables and matricellular proteins. The proteins osteopontin, periostin, and galectin-3 had prediction accuracies of 95.1%, 78.1%, and 3.8%, respectively. These studies demonstrate that ML methods have shown excellent performance in predicting complications that arise from aneurysm rupture.

Another application is the use of clinical data and CT perfusion from hospital admissions to predict outcomes of aneurysmal SAH. A random forest model was trained to predict dichotomized mRS (<2 and >2), and the accuracy was 84.4% in the training folds and 70.9% in the validation folds. However, it cannot be introduced into clinical practice because of small population size [50].

5. Limitations and challenges of AI on intracranial aneurysm

The use of artificial intelligence in the analysis of intracranial aneurysms has been expanding rapidly. While numerous algorithms and techniques have been developed for managing these aneurysms, certain challenges and limitations must be addressed.

Kim and colleagues [51] suggested certain standards to assess the clinical effectiveness of AI algorithms. These include obtaining external validation, conducting a diagnostic cohort study, involving multiple institutions, and performing prospective studies. However, most of the studies on AI in managing intracranial aneurysms lack external validation and are retrospectively designed, which can lead to selection bias and variability. To achieve reliable results, it is necessary to conduct prospective studies and externally validate the available algorithms for their clinical feasibility [5].

DL-based algorithms have exhibited positive outcomes, along with other AI techniques. However, the time taken to train them and their cost-effectiveness are still questionable. The intricate structure of neural network algorithms poses a challenge known as the "black box" problem, where the process of data processing within the layers is not completely understood. This leads to skepticism regarding the results generated from a "black box" [19].

In addition, these systems may introduce new kinds of errors, particularly automation bias, which is defined as the inclination to use automated cues as a substitute for vigilant information-seeking and processing [52]. Automation bias has been highlighted as one of the potential drawbacks and ethical issues of AI-based applications. It reflects the dependence of the user on the machine, ignoring the contradictory information that may exist without automation, leading to decreased self-confidence and loss of human input [5].

Nowadays, a legal consensus is lacking regarding AI regulations, and no clear guidelines are available regarding the independent mathematical interrogation and validation of outputs generated by AI systems [52].

6. Future perspectives

AI has promising potential in the management of intracranial aneurysms in the future, including prescreening triage systems for emergency medicine physicians to prioritize high-risk patients, automated detection and intelligent outcome prediction, prediction of treatment strategies during follow-up, automated detection of recurrence after treatment, and prediction of rupture risk [1].

For an AI tool to effectively manage aneurysms, it must accurately identify true-positive cases with high confidence. This level of reliability can only be achieved through a significant number of annotated imaging studies, which are necessary before the tool can be widely implemented in real-world scenarios [53].

7. Conclusions

In conclusion, the use of artificial intelligence in managing intracranial aneurysms offers higher accuracy and efficacy than manual measurements and can potentially augment the clinical performance of radiologists and shorten interpretation time. While some studies need to be validated in a clinical setting, AI-based applications should be viewed as a tool to assist and not replace human decision-making in health care. Although implementing new technology may initially be costly, the long-term cost-effectiveness of AI can potentially reduce the cost of unnecessary diagnostic testing. Further studies are required to explore other AI applications in intracranial aneurysms and to validate the findings in a real-world clinical setting.

Acknowledgements

This work would not have been possible without the financial support of Fundación Amigos de la Juventud, A.C. (FUNDAJU).

Conflict of interest

The authors declare no conflict of interest.

Author details

Luis Antonio Marín-Castañeda, Fernanda de Leon-Mendoza
and Hector Eduardo Valdez-Ruvalcaba*
Stroke Clinic, National Institute of Neurology and Neurosurgery, Mexico City, Mexico

*Address all correspondence to: dr.valdez.neurologia@gmail.com

References

[1] Shi Z, Hu B, Schoepf UJ, Savage RH, Dargis DM, Pan CW, et al. Artificial intelligence in the management of intracranial aneurysms: Current status and future perspectives. American Journal of Neuroradiology. 2020;**41**(3):373-379

[2] Vlak MH, Algra A, Brandenburg R, Rinkel GJ. Prevalence of unruptured intracranial aneurysms, with emphasis on sex, age, comorbidity, country, and time period: A systematic review and meta-analysis. Lancet Neurology. 2011;**10**(7):626-636

[3] Turan N, Heider RA, Roy AK, Miller BA, Mullins ME, Barrow DL, et al. Current perspectives in imaging modalities for the assessment of unruptured intracranial aneurysms: A comparative analysis and review. World Neurosurgery. 2018;**113**:280-292

[4] Yoon NK, McNally S, Taussky P, Park MS. Imaging of cerebral aneurysms: A clinical perspective. Neurovascular Imaging. 2016;**2**(1):6

[5] Alwalid O, Long X, Xie M, Han P. Artificial intelligence applications in intracranial aneurysm: Achievements, challenges and opportunities. Academic Radiology. 2022;**29**:S201-S214

[6] Etminan N, Brown RD, Beseoglu K, Juvela S, Raymond J, Morita A, et al. The unruptured intracranial aneurysm treatment score. Neurology. 2015;**85**(10):881-889

[7] Andresen SL. John McCarthy: Father of AI. IEEE Intelligent Systems. 2002;**17**(5):84-85

[8] Staartjes VE, Regli L, Serra C. Machine intelligence in clinical neuroscience: Taming the unchained. Prometheus. 2022;**2022**:1-4

[9] Yin J, Ngiam KY, Teo HH. Role of artificial intelligence applications in real-life clinical practice: Systematic review. Journal of Medical Internet Research. 2021;**23**(4):e25759

[10] Massaad E, Ha Y, Shankar GM, Shin JH. Clinical prediction modeling in intramedullary spinal tumor surgery. Machine Learning in Clinical Neuroscience 2022:333-339

[11] Swinburne NC, Schefflein J, Sakai Y, Oermann EK, Titano JJ, Chen I, et al. Machine learning for semiautomated classification of glioblastoma, brain metastasis and central nervous system lymphoma using magnetic resonance advanced imaging. Annals of Translational Medicine. 2019;**7**(11):232-232

[12] Varatharajah Y, Berry B, Cimbalnik J, Kremen V, van Gompel J, Stead M, et al. Integrating artificial intelligence with real-time intracranial EEG monitoring to automate interictal identification of seizure onset zones in focal epilepsy. Journal of Neural Engineering. 2018;**15**(4):046035

[13] Carcagnì P, Leo M, del Coco M, Distante C, de Salve A. Convolution neural networks and self-attention learners for Alzheimer dementia diagnosis from brain MRI. Sensors. 2023;**23**(3):1694

[14] Shalaby A, Soliman A, Elaskary S, Refaey A, Abdelazim M, Khalifa F. Editorial: Artificial intelligence based computer-aided diagnosis applications for brain disorders from medical imaging data. Frontiers in Neuroscience. 2023;**31**:17

[15] English M, Kumar C, Ditterline BL, Drazin D, Dietz N. Machine learning in neuro-oncology, epilepsy. Alzheimer's Disease, and Schizophrenia. 2022:349-361

[16] Jin MC, Rodrigues AJ, Jensen M, Veeravagu A. A discussion of machine learning approaches for clinical prediction. Modeling. 2022;**2022**:65-73

[17] Mintz Y, Brodie R. Introduction to artificial intelligence in medicine. Minimally Invasive Therapy and Allied Technologies. 2019;**28**(2):73-81

[18] Millan RD, Dempere-Marco L, Pozo JM, Cebral JR, Frangi AF. Morphological characterization of intracranial aneurysms using 3-D moment invariants. IEEE Transactions on Medical Imaging. 2007;**26**(9):1270-1282

[19] Mensah E, Pringle C, Roberts G, Gurusinghe N, Golash A, Alalade AF. Deep learning in the management of intracranial aneurysms and cerebrovascular diseases: A review of the current literature. World Neurosurgery. 2022;**161**:39-45

[20] Arimura H, Li Q, Korogi Y, Hirai T, Abe H, Yamashita Y, et al. Automated computerized scheme for detection of unruptured intracranial aneurysms in three-dimensional magnetic resonance angiography1. Academic Radiology. 2004;**11**(10):1093-1104

[21] Yang X, Blezek DJ, Cheng LTE, Ryan WJ, Kallmes DF, Erickson BJ. Computer-aided detection of intracranial aneurysms in MR angiography. Journal of Digital Imaging. 2011;**24**(1):86-95

[22] Bo ZH, Qiao H, Tian C, Guo Y, Li W, Liang T, et al. Toward human intervention-free clinical diagnosis of intracranial aneurysm via deep neural network. Patterns. 2021;**2**(2):100197

[23] Joo B, Choi HS, Ahn SS, Cha J, Won SY, Sohn B, et al. A deep learning model with high standalone performance for diagnosis of unruptured intracranial aneurysm. Yonsei Medical Journal. 2021;**62**(11):1052

[24] Shi Z, Miao C, Schoepf UJ, Savage RH, Dargis DM, Pan C, et al. A clinically applicable deep-learning model for detecting intracranial aneurysm in computed tomography angiography images. Nature Communications. 2020;**11**(1):6090

[25] Sichtermann T, Faron A, Sijben R, Teichert N, Freiherr J, Wiesmann M. Deep learning–based detection of intracranial aneurysms in 3D TOF-MRA. American Journal of Neuroradiology. 2019;**40**(1):25-32

[26] Stember JN, Chang P, Stember DM, Liu M, Grinband J, Filippi CG, et al. Convolutional neural networks for the detection and measurement of cerebral aneurysms on magnetic resonance angiography. Journal of Digital Imaging. 2019;**32**(5):808-815

[27] Ueda D, Yamamoto A, Nishimori M, Shimono T, Doishita S, Shimazaki A, et al. Deep learning for MR angiography: Automated detection of cerebral aneurysms. Radiology. 2019;**290**(1):187-194

[28] Nakao T, Hanaoka S, Nomura Y, Sato I, Nemoto M, Miki S, et al. Deep neural network-based computer-assisted detection of cerebral aneurysms in MR angiography. Journal of Magnetic Resonance Imaging. 2018;**47**(4):948-953

[29] Park A, Chute C, Rajpurkar P, Lou J, Ball RL, Shpanskaya K, et al. Deep learning–assisted diagnosis of

cerebral aneurysms using the HeadXNet model. JAMA Network Open. 2019;**2**(6):e195600

[30] Yang J, Xie M, Hu C, Alwalid O, Xu Y, Liu J, et al. Deep learning for detecting cerebral aneurysms with CT angiography. Radiology. 2021;**298**(1):155-163

[31] Jin H, Geng J, Yin Y, Hu M, Yang G, Xiang S, et al. Fully automated intracranial aneurysm detection and segmentation from digital subtraction angiography series using an end-to-end spatiotemporal deep neural network. Journal of Neurointervention Surgery. 2020;**12**(10):1023-1027

[32] Duan H, Huang Y, Liu L, Dai H, Chen L, Zhou L. Automatic detection on intracranial aneurysm from digital subtraction angiography with cascade convolutional neural networks. Biomedical Engineering Online. 2019;**18**(1):110

[33] Pierot L, Wakhloo AK. Endovascular treatment of intracranial aneurysms. Stroke. 2013;**44**(7):2046-2054

[34] Velagapudi L, Saiegh F, Swaminathan S, Mouchtouris N, Khanna O, Sabourin V, et al. Machine learning for outcome prediction of neurosurgical aneurysm treatment: Current methods and future directions. Clinical Neurology and Neurosurgery. 2023;**224**:107547

[35] Marasini A, Shrestha A, Phuyal S, Zaidat OO, Kalia JS. Role of artificial intelligence in unruptured intracranial aneurysm: An overview. Frontiers in Neurology. 2022;**23**:13

[36] Choudhri O, Mukerji N, Steinberg GK. Combined endovascular and microsurgical management of complex cerebral aneurysms. Frontiers in Neurology. 2013;**2013**:4

[37] Barker FG, Amin-Hanjani S, Butler WE, Ogilvy CS, Carter BS. In-hospital mortality and morbidity after surgical treatment of unruptured intracranial aneurysms in the United States, 1996-2000: The effect of hospital and surgeon volume. Neurosurgery. 2003;**52**(5):995-1009

[38] Iqbal J, Jahangir K, Mashkoor Y, Sultana N, Mehmood D, Ashraf M, et al. The future of artificial intelligence in neurosurgery: A narrative review. Surgical Neurology International. 2022;**13**:536

[39] Dovey Z, Misra M, Thornton J, Charbel FT, Debrun GM, Ausman JI. Guglielmi detachable coiling for intracranial aneurysms: The story so far. Archives of Neurology. 2001;**58**(4):559-564

[40] Brinjikji W, Murad MH, Lanzino G, Cloft HJ, Kallmes DF. Endovascular treatment of intracranial aneurysms with flow diverters. Stroke. 2013;**44**(2):442-447

[41] Xiang J, Antiga L, Varble N, Snyder K, Levy EI, Siddiqui AH, et al. A view: An image-based clinical computational tool for intracranial aneurysm flow visualization and clinical management. Annals of Biomedical Engineering. 2016;**44**(4):1085-1096

[42] Xiang J, Damiano RJ, Lin N, Snyder K, Siddiqui AH, Levy EI, et al. High-fidelity virtual stenting: Modeling of flow diverter deployment for hemodynamic characterization of complex intracranial aneurysms. Journal of Neurosurgery. 2015;**123**(4):832-840

[43] Mut F, Raschi M, Scrivano E, Bleise C, Chudyk J, Ceratto R, et al. Association between hemodynamic conditions and occlusion times after

flow diversion in cerebral aneurysms. Journal of Neurointervention Surgery. 2015;7(4):286-290

[44] Paliwal N, Jaiswal P, Tutino VM, Shallwani H, Davies JM, Siddiqui AH, et al. Outcome prediction of intracranial aneurysm treatment by flow diverters using machine learning. Neurosurgical Focus. 2018;**45**(5):E7

[45] Guédon A, Thépenier C, Shotar E, Gabrieli J, Mathon B, Premat K, et al. Predictive score for complete occlusion of intracranial aneurysms treated by flow-diverter stents using machine learning. Journal of Neurointervention Surgery. 2021;**13**(4):341-346

[46] Zhu W, Li W, Tian Z, Zhang Y, Wang K, Zhang Y, et al. Stability assessment of intracranial aneurysms using machine learning based on clinical and morphological features. Translational Stroke Research. 2020;**11**(6):1287-1295

[47] Tanioka S, Ishida F, Yamamoto A, Shimizu S, Sakaida H, Toyoda M, et al. Machine learning classification of cerebral aneurysm rupture status with morphologic variables and hemodynamic parameters. Radiological Artificial Intelligence. 2020;**2**(1):e190077

[48] Savarraj JPJ, Hergenroeder GW, Zhu L, Chang T, Park S, Megjhani M, et al. Machine learning to predict delayed cerebral ischemia and outcomes in subarachnoid Hemorrhage. Neurology. 2021;**96**(4):e553-e562

[49] Dumont TM, Rughani AI, Tranmer BI. Prediction of symptomatic cerebral vasospasm after aneurysmal subarachnoid hemorrhage with an artificial neural network: Feasibility and comparison with logistic regression models. World Neurosurgery. 2011;**75**(1):57-63

[50] Rubbert C, Patil KR, Beseoglu K, Mathys C, May R, Kaschner MG, et al. Prediction of outcome after aneurysmal subarachnoid haemorrhage using data from patient admission. European Radiology. 2018;**28**(12):4949-4958

[51] Kim DW, Jang HY, Kim KW, Shin Y, Park SH. Design characteristics of studies reporting the performance of artificial intelligence algorithms for diagnostic analysis of medical images: Results from recently published papers. Korean Journal of Radiology. 2019;**20**(3):405

[52] Lyell D, Coiera E. Automation bias and verification complexity: A systematic review. Journal of the American Medical Informatics Association. 2017;**24**(2):423-431

[53] Hesamian MH, Jia W, He X, Kennedy P. Deep learning techniques for medical image segmentation: Achievements and challenges. Journal of Digital Imaging. 2019;**32**(4):582-596

Chapter 4

Clinical Application of Transcranial Doppler in Cerebrovascular Diseases

Michelle P. Lin

Abstract

Transcranial doppler (TCD) ultrasonography is a diagnostic technology for ascertaining numerous physiologic and pathologic phenomena by monitoring the direction and velocity of blood flow in intracranial vasculature. It is a noninvasive, point-of-care diagnostic tool that provides continuous and reproducible bedside data without the use of radiation or contrast agents. In this chapter, we will review principles TCD ultrasonography, and review clinical utility of TCD in aneurysmal subarachnoid hemorrhage (aSAH) and stroke as relate TCD monitoring. We will also review the advances in the clinical application of TCD in cerebrovascular diseases including robotic assisted TCD devices in PFO detection as well as clinical trials using TCD for early detection of large-vessel occlusive ischemic stroke.

Keywords: transcranial doppler, aneurysmal subarachnoid hemorrhage, ischemic stroke, aneurysm, treatment

1. Introduction

Transcranial doppler (TCD) is a non-invasive ultrasound technique that allows for the assessment of cerebral blood flow velocity in real-time without the use of iodine radiation commonly used in neurocritical care. It is an important bedside tool in the evaluation of cerebrovascular diseases including aneurysmal subarachnoid hemorrhage (aSAH) and ischemic stroke. In this chapter, we will review the principles of transcranial doppler, and the clinical application of TCD in aSAH for monitoring vasospasm and microemboli detection in large-vessel vasculopathy. We will also review the advances in the clinical application of TCD in cerebrovascular diseases robotic assisted TCD devices in PFO detection as well as clinical trials using TCD for early detection of large-vessel occlusive ischemic stroke.

2. Transcranial Doppler principles

The *Doppler effect* is the shift in frequency emitted by a source moving in relation to an observer as perceived by the observer. The shift is to higher frequencies when the distance between the source and the observer decreases and to lower frequencies when the distance increases. In TCD, the source is a red blood cell reflecting an echo, and the observer is the ultrasound probe.

TCD instruments are generally calibrated to measure blood flow velocity when blood is moving either directly toward the ultrasound probe (0°) or directly away from it (180°). This principle is important because if insonation is at an angle other than 0° or 180°, only a fraction of the true velocity is measured. Certain areas on and around the skull (*windows of insonation*) help the operator achieve insonation directly in line with blood flow and avoid signal attenuation from the skull and other tissue. **Figure 1** shows TCD acoustic windows. The arteries that are examined at those windows are as follows:

- Transtemporal window: MCA, anterior cerebral artery (ACA), terminal portion of the internal carotid artery (ICA), and posterior cerebral artery (PCA).
- Transorbital (ophthalmic) window: ophthalmic artery and ICA at the siphon level.
- Submandibular window: distal portion of the extracranial ICA.
- Transforaminal (occipital) window: basilar artery (BA) and vertebral artery (VA).

Temporal window is commonly accessed as it provides optimal visualization of MCA, which is frequently involved artery in stroke. Temporal window is an areas of the skull that is located just above the zygomatic arch, approximately 1 cm posterior to the midpoint of a line connecting the lateral canthus of the eye to the auditory

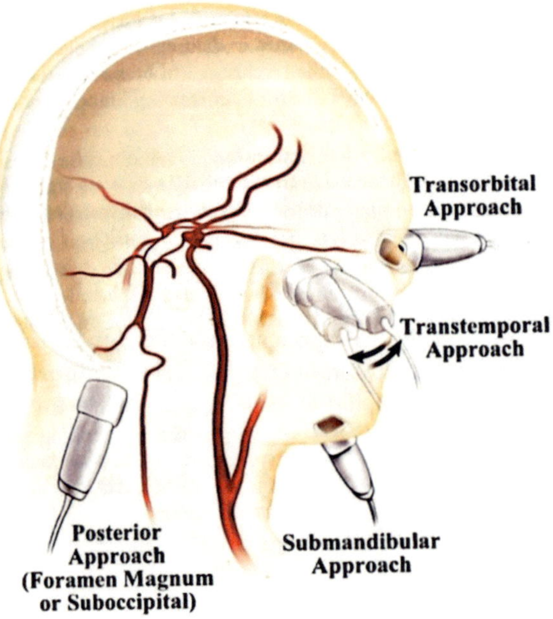

Figure 1.
TCD acoustic windows.

meatus. The ultrasound probe is positioned on the temporal bone and angled to obtain a transcranial view of the MCA. This allows for detection of emboli, stenosis, and changes in blood flow velocity that may indicate cerebral ischemia or Vasospasm.

An understanding of cerebral hemodynamics, including relevant anatomy, physiology, and pathophysiology, is critical for the accurate acquisition and interpretation of intracranial Doppler data. To this end, it is important to understand the typical vascular distributions and the manifold factors that can affect cerebral blood flow. The cerebral vasculature has autoregulatory mechanisms that compensate for changes in cardiac output and blood viscosity, thereby maintaining relatively constant cerebral blood flow (and cerebral blood flow velocity as measured with TCD). Nevertheless, extreme changes in hemostasis will affect cerebral blood flow. For example, in larger arteries, atherosclerotic plaques cause arterial stenosis alters blood flow velocity. In smaller arteries, various precipitants (e.g., arterial carbon dioxide, intracranial pressure, and mean arterial pressure) alter the flow, and the upstream effects can be inferred from TCD.

3. TCD in aneurysmal subarachnoid hemorrhage

Aneurysmal subarachnoid hemorrhage is a life-threatening condition that can result in significant morbidity and mortality. Vasospasm and delayed cerebral ischemia (DCI) are common complication of aSAH; they contribute to substantial morbidity and mortality after aSAH [1]. TCD can detect vasospasm by measuring changes in cerebral blood flow velocity with daily monitoring. A study found that TCD had high sensitivity and specificity in detecting vasospasm in aSAH patients [2]. DCI is another common complication of aSAH that can lead to poor outcomes. DCI is thought to be caused by vasospasm from endothelial dysfunction and microthrombosis [3, 4]. TCD can detect changes in cerebral blood flow velocity and microemboli associated with DCI to determine the appropriate timing of intervention such as intraarterial or oral calcium channel blockers to treat vasospasm in aSAH [5].

TCD measures blood flow velocity in all vessels in the circle-of-Willis, but especially for the MCA. Trends in the baseline TCD mean flow velocity (MFV) over time in patients with SAH are recommended for screening for vasospasm. MFV is most sensitive and specific for angiographic vasospasm in the MCA, whereas it is less sensitive and specific for the first segments of the ACA and PCA.

The Lindegaard ratio (or the hemispheric ratio) is the ratio of the MCA flow velocity to the ipsilateral ICA flow velocity. The ratio is often used in conjunction with MCA MFV and accounts for hemodynamic augmentation from a hyperdynamic state (e.g., from pressors or an endogenous hypersympathetic state). A Lindegaard ratio less than 3 suggests a hyperdynamic state with potential relative vasospasm as defined according to the MCA MFV (MCA MFV >120 cm/s indicates mild vasospasm; >150 cm/s, moderate; and >200 cm/s, severe). A Lindegaard ratio greater than 3 typically correlates with angiographic vasospasm seen on computed tomographic angiography (CTA) (>180 cm/s with perfusion impairment); a ratio greater than 6 indicates a high-grade angiographic spasm that may warrant an endovascular neurosurgery consultation.

With established normative data, TCD can be used to compare extracranial and intracranial flow velocities to help localize an intracranial stenosis as distinguished from a hyperdynamic state that is increasing the blood flow velocity (Lindegaard ratio = MCA flow velocity/distal extracranial ICA flow velocity; Soustiel ratio = BA flow velocity/distal extracranial VA flow velocity). Velocity trends are checked in each vessel daily and correlated with symptoms or radiographic spasm as a noninvasive means of investigating the "spasm window." Velocities usually increase in the first 3 days after bleeding and decrease at 9–14 days. All these provide daily monitoring of cerebral and systemic hemodynamics to guide optimal aSAH treatments.

While TCD is non-invasive, bedside procedure without need for contrast or radiation, it has several limitations. First, it is operator-dependent and often limited from craniotomy wound. Second, TCD correlates well with angiographic vasospasm but not necessarily with symptomatic vasospasm (i.e., clinical deficits). Many confounders are related to the systemic illness associated with aneurysmal SAH: increased ICP, hemodynamic instability, changes in $PaCO_2$ or hematocrit, and collateralization. Despite these limitations, combining with other multimodal neuromonitoring for vasospasm and DCI, TCD adds tremendous value to the management of aneurysmal subarachnoid hemorrhage.

4. TCD in stroke for emboli detection

Stroke is a major cause of morbidity and mortality worldwide. Early detection and treatment are crucial for improving outcomes in stroke patients. TCD has been used as a diagnostic tool to evaluate cerebral blood flow changes or microembolic in stroke patients to guide treatments. TCD can detect the presence of distal emboli from proximal intracranial or extracranial arterial stenosis or occlusions, and it can also monitor changes in cerebral blood flow velocity and wave form patterns during and after thrombolytic therapy for response and prognosticate outcomes.

In cervical carotid stenosis, several studies have shown that TCD can detect embolic signals in the middle cerebral artery, which is the most commonly affected site in carotid artery disease [6, 7]. Markus et al. found that asymptomatic cerebral emboli signals, high-intensity transient signals (HITS), were present in 58% of patients with symptomatic carotid artery disease and in 37% of patients with asymptomatic disease [6]. Same group also demonstrated asymptomatic cerebral emboli detection over 1 h in 200 patients with >50% symptomatic carotid stenosis was associated with 4.67-fold increased risk of recurrent ipsilateral ischemic events in adjusted cox regression model [7]. TCD is also utilized in predicting risk of stroke in patients with high-risk plaque features such as intraplaque hemorrhage. Sitzer et al. reported that plaque ulceration and lumen thrombus are the main sources of cerebral microemboli in high-grade internal carotid artery stenosis [8]. TCD can be used during carotid endarterectomy to detect emboli in real-time and guide the surgeon to take appropriate measures to prevent embolic events. Spencer et al. demonstrated that TCD could detect middle cerebral artery emboli during carotid endarterectomy, with a sensitivity of 92% and a specificity of 100% [9]. Therefore, TCD is a useful tool in the detection of cerebral emboli in carotid stenosis, which can help guide decision for intervention and surgical approach to minimize risk of stroke.

5. TCD for cerebrovascular reactivity

Cerebrovascular reserve (CVR) is the ability of brain to autoregulate cerebral blood flow in response to physiologic changes such as arterial occlusion as in stroke. Impaired CV in patients with steno-occlusive disease is associated with increased risk of stroke [10–12]. CVR quantified change in cerebral blood flow in response to vasodilatory stimuli such as carbon dioxide (CO2). Several multiple modalities for measuring CVR, including Blood Oxygen Level Dependent (BOLD) or arterial spin labeling (ASL) MR imaging with CO2 challenge, CT perfusion with acetazolamide. Among these noninvasive modalities, TCD is the most commonly used modality for assessing CVR and guiding decisions for revascularization. A systematic review involving 754 patients with asympatomic severe carotid stenosis and impaired CVR on TCD had 3.69 fold increased risk of ipsilateral ischemic stroke (HR 3.69, 95% CI 2.01–6.77, $P < 0.001$) [11].

CVR measured by TCD appears to be a useful tool for predicting outcomes after revascularization in patients with carotid stenosis or ICAD. However, due to the dynamic and time-variant nature of CVR, the influence of aging (normal or pathologic aging), exposure to common vasoactive agents such as caffefine or medications, and diurnal variation on CVR in relationship to cerebrovascular diseases is not yet well understood.

A recent study involving 185 healthy adults between the age of 21 and 80 years, who underwent TCD and multimodal MRI, revealed that blood flow velocity decreases with age while the caliber of large vessels remains similar among age groups. These findings suggest that age-related decreases in CBFV and impaired CVR likely reflect small vessel diseases [13]. Another study further demonstrated that the speed of CVR of MCA response to induced vasodilation with CO_2 slowed with age [14]. Further research is needed to gain a deeper understanding of the implications of CVR on treatment decisions and to determine optimal threshold values for CVR across all age groups, enabling informed therapeutic decisions.

6. TCD for PFO detection

Right to left shunt from patent foramen ovale (PFO) is a common anatomical variation in which there is an opening between the right and left atria, and it can be a potential risk factor for cryptogenic stroke [15]. Several randomized clinical trials support closure of PFO in patients between age 16 and 60 years who suffer from cryptogenic stroke from paradoxical embolism through PFO. TCD can detect microbubbles that cross from the right to the left atrium during a Valsalva maneuver, indicating the presence of a PFO. A meta-analysis by Mojadidi et al. showed that TCD has a sensitivity of 97% and a specificity of 93% for the detection of PFO compared to transesophageal echocardiography, which is the gold standard imaging modality for PFO detection [16]. However, TCD is less invasive and less expensive than TEE, making it an attractive alternative for PFO detection in certain patient populations. In addition, TCD can be performed at the bedside, allowing for real-time evaluation of PFO during a Valsalva maneuver, which can provide valuable information about the hemodynamic significance of the PFO in stroke pathogenesis. Overall, TCD is a reliable and cost-effective tool for the detection of PFO in patients with cryptogenic stroke.

While TCD is very sensitivity and specific for the detection of PFO, it relies heavily on the operator's technical skills and availability of trained technicians. Recently, a robotic-assistant TCD (ra-TCD) system with artificial intelligence (AI)-enhanced signal detection algorithms has been tested in clinical research to mitigate the variability in TCD acquisition. The BUBL study is a multicenter, prospective trial comparing raTCD to TTE for PFO detection (NCT04604015) [17]. The study found that raTCD detecting all and large RLS at approximately three times the rate of TTE (primary outcome, any RLS: raTCD 64% vs. TTE 20% [absolute difference 43.4% (95% CI 34.3–52.5%), $p < 0.001$]) [18]. Ongoing studies are testing whether these results are generalizable in routine practice.

7. Conclusion

TCD is a non-invasive ultrasound technique that allows for the assessment of cerebral blood flow velocity in real-time. It has emerged as an important diagnostic tool in the evaluation of cerebrovascular diseases such as aSAH and ischemic stroke. TCD can detect cerebral blood flow changes that can help guide clinical management and improve patient outcomes. TCD has been used to diagnose and monitor changes in cerebral blood flow velocity in stroke patients, and to detect vasospasm and DCI in aSAH patients. TCD can also guide treatment decisions in these patients. Further research is needed to determine the full extent of the utility of TCD in these conditions.

Goals

- Review the principles of transcranial Doppler (TCD) ultrasonography.
- Review the clinical utility of TCD in monitoring vasospasm after aneurysmal subarachnoid hemorrhage.
- Review the clinical utility of TCD in ischemic stroke including microemboli and PFO detections, and cerebrovascular reactivity quantification.

Author details

Michelle P. Lin
Department of Neurology, Mayo Clinic, Jacksonville, FL, United States

*Address all correspondence to: lin.michelle@mayo.edu

References

[1] Chou SH. Subarachnoid hemorrhage. Continuum (Minneap Minn). 2021;**27**:1201-1245

[2] Sloan MA, Haley EC Jr, Kassell NF, Henry ML, Stewart SR, Beskin RR, et al. Sensitivity and specificity of transcranial doppler ultrasonography in the diagnosis of vasospasm following subarachnoid hemorrhage. Neurology. 1989;**39**:1514-1518

[3] Vergouwen MD, Vermeulen M, van Gijn J, Rinkel GJ, Wijdicks EF, Muizelaar JP, et al. Definition of delayed cerebral ischemia after aneurysmal subarachnoid hemorrhage as an outcome event in clinical trials and observational studies: Proposal of a multidisciplinary research group. Stroke. 2010;**41**:2391-2395

[4] Sehba FA, Pluta RM, Zhang JH. Metamorphosis of subarachnoid hemorrhage research: From delayed vasospasm to early brain injury. Molecular Neurobiology. 2011;**43**:27-40

[5] de Rooij NK, Rinkel GJ, Dankbaar JW, Frijns CJ. Delayed cerebral ischemia after subarachnoid hemorrhage: A systematic review of clinical, laboratory, and radiological predictors. Stroke. 2013;**44**:43-54

[6] Markus HS, Thomson ND, Brown MM. Asymptomatic cerebral embolic signals in symptomatic and asymptomatic carotid artery disease. Brain. 1995;**118**(Pt 4):1005-1011

[7] Markus HS, MacKinnon A. Asymptomatic embolization detected by doppler ultrasound predicts stroke risk in symptomatic carotid artery stenosis. Stroke. 2005;**36**:971-975

[8] Sitzer M, Müller W, Siebler M, Hort W, Kniemeyer HW, Jäncke L, et al. Plaque ulceration and lumen thrombus are the main sources of cerebral microemboli in high-grade internal carotid artery stenosis. Stroke. 1995;**26**:1231-1233

[9] Spencer MP, Thomas GI, Nicholls SC, Sauvage LR. Detection of middle cerebral artery emboli during carotid endarterectomy using transcranial doppler ultrasonography. Stroke. 1990;**21**:415-423

[10] Vernieri F, Pasqualetti P, Passarelli F, Rossini PM, Silvestrini M. Outcome of carotid artery occlusion is predicted by cerebrovascular reactivity. Stroke. 1999;**30**:593-598

[11] Reinhard M, Schwarzer G, Briel M, Altamura C, Palazzo P, King A, et al. Cerebrovascular reactivity predicts stroke in high-grade carotid artery disease. Neurology. 2014;**83**:1424-1431

[12] Silvestrini M, Vernieri F, Pasqualetti P, Matteis M, Passarelli F, Troisi E, et al. Impaired cerebral vasoreactivity and risk of stroke in patients with asymptomatic carotid artery stenosis. Journal of the American Medical Association. 2000;**283**:2122-2127

[13] Tomoto T, Lu M, Khan AM, Liu J, Pasha EP, Tarumi T, et al. Cerebral blood flow and cerebrovascular resistance across the adult lifespan: A multimodality approach. Journal of Cerebral Blood Flow and Metabolism. 2023;**2023**:271678x231153741

[14] Koep JL, Bond B, Barker AR, Ruediger SL, Pizzey FK, Coombes JS, et al. The relationships between age, sex, and cerebrovascular reactivity to hypercapnia using traditional and kinetic-based analyses in healthy

adults. American Journal of Physiology. Heart and Circulatory Physiology. 2022;**323**:H782-h796

[15] Mazzucco S, Li L, Binney L, Rothwell PM. Prevalence of patent foramen ovale in cryptogenic transient ischaemic attack and non-disabling stroke at older ages: A population-based study, systematic review, and meta-analysis. Lancet Neurology. 2018;**17**:609-617

[16] Mojadidi MK, Roberts SC, Winoker JS, Romero J, Goodman-Meza D, Gevorgyan R, et al. Accuracy of transcranial doppler for the diagnosis of intracardiac right-to-left shunt: A bivariate meta-analysis of prospective studies. JACC: Cardiovascular Imaging. 2014;7:236-250

[17] Rubin MN, Alexandrov AV, Douville C, Rinsky B, Tsivgoulis G. Novel robotic tcd ultrasound with bubbles versus standard care to detect right to left shunt: Study methods. Journal of Neuroimaging. 2021;**31**:858-863

[18] Rubin M. Robotic tcd ultrasound bubble study compared to transthoracic echocardiography for detection of right to left shunt (bubl). In: An Abstract Presented at the 2022 International Stroke Conference in New Orleans. 2022

Section 2

Operative Management

Chapter 5

Keyhole Microsurgery for Cerebral Aneurysms

Revaz Dzhindzhikhadze, Renat Kambiev, Andrey Polyakov, Andrey Zaitsev, Anton Ermolaev and Igor Bogdanovich

Abstract

The choice of an effective and safe surgical approach is an important and largely outcome-determining step in the microsurgical treatment of cerebral aneurysms. Transcranial approach to aneurysm should provide proximal and distal control, visualization of the aneurysm and surrounding structures, freedom to work with microinstruments, optimal and close view of the surgical field with the necessary ergonomics and the possibility of comfortable work for the neurosurgeon. In addition, the approach should provide a low risk of associated complications, good cosmetic outcomes and patient satisfaction. Today, a neurosurgeon has a sufficient number of approaches to cerebral aneurysms. Minimally invasive approaches are the reduced model of traditional approaches and each of these approaches has a specific surgical corridor that cannot be changed during microsurgical manipulations, unless through the transition to an extended craniotomy.

Keywords: keyhole, cerebral aneurysms, supraorbital approach, transorbital approach, microsurgery

1. Introduction

The rapid development of minimally invasive neurosurgery is associated with the wide availability and distribution of highly informative neuroimaging technologies. Neurosurgeons often face the problem of choosing the most optimal treatment method in search of minimizing surgical aggression. For several decades, in the surgical treatment of aneurysms, pterional craniotomy has been the traditional approach for most aneurysms of the anterior parts of the cerebral arterial circle and the upper parts of the basilar artery [1]. However, upon critical analysis, it becomes clear that the "collateral damage" of tissues during craniotomy is not related to the immediate goal of the surgical intervention. These negative consequences affect the immediate and long-term recovery of patients and prolonged hospitalization, which leads to long-term disability and, accordingly, economic costs.

The popularization of the concept of "keyhole" surgery is associated with the possibility of accurate preoperative planning, improvement of microneurosurgical techniques, intraoperative control in the form of fluorescein angiography, video endoscopic assistance and neurophysiological monitoring, which allows focusing on the accuracy,

IntechOpen

efficiency, and safety of surgical intervention. It is important that minimally invasive approaches make it possible to minimize iatrogenic trauma by creating an individual surgical corridor. The principle of "individual" access to cerebral aneurysms is reduced to the use of several minimally invasive approaches depending on the specific neuro-imaging pattern in comparison with the previously used algorithm and the choice of pterional craniotomy for all aneurysms of the anterior cerebral arterial circle [2–7].

The modern concept of microsurgical treatment of cerebral aneurysms involves the choice of an individual approach. The main goal of individualization is to create the shortest efficient route to the target with minimal collateral damage, ensuring the safety of the intervention. Individualized minimally invasive approach in the microsurgical treatment of cerebral aneurysms improves surgical and clinical outcomes, reduces the time of surgery, length of stay in the hospital, and the cost of treatment and provides excellent cosmetic results [4, 6, 7].

The three keyhole approaches are discussed below: eyebrow supraorbital, minipterional and transorbitals.

2. Types of keyhole approaches

Minimally invasive approaches are reduced models of traditional craniotomies: pterional, supraorbital, orbitozygomatic, etc. (**Figure 1**).

2.1 Eyebrow supraorbital approach (ESA)

Supraorbital craniotomy with a skin incision through the eyebrow is an anterolateral surgical route that provides access to the aneurysms of the anterior circulation and the upper basilar artery [5, 6, 8–10]. Main indications for ESA:

- Anterior circulation aneurysms
- Internal carotid artery (ICA)

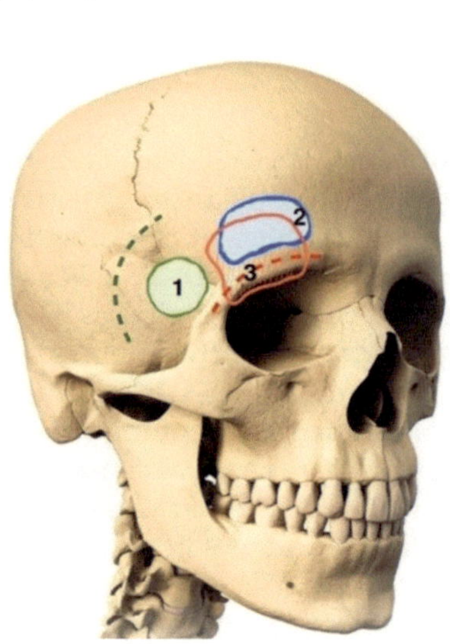

Figure 1.
Types of minimally invasive approaches. 1 - minipterional, 2 - eyebrow supraorbital, 3 - eyebrow transorbital.

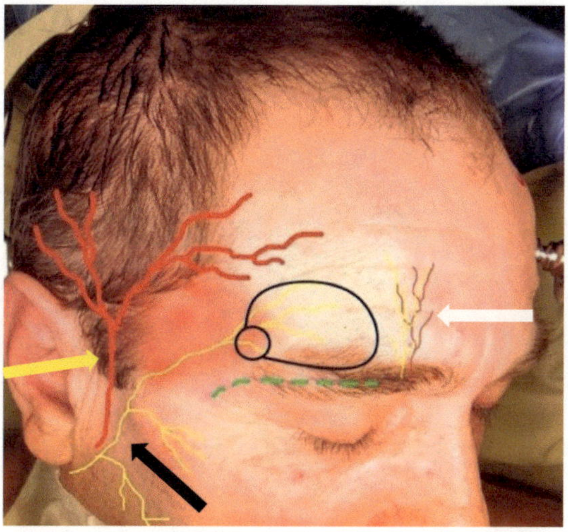

Figure 2.
Intraoperative photograph. Schematic representation of the main anatomical landmarks of ESA. Bone borders are marked in black. The skin incision is marked in green. Arrows: white - supraorbital nerve and artery, black - branches of the facial nerve, yellow - superficial temporal artery.

- Anterior cerebral artery (ACA) A1-A2 segments
- Anterior communicating artery (Acom)
- Middle cerebral artery (MCA) M1 segment-M2 segments (if M1 segment is not more than 20 mm)

Anatomical landmarks assessed for EAS:

- supraorbital notch,
- superior margin of the orbit,
- and superior temporal line,
- the topography of the frontal sinuses is preliminarily assessed based on neuroimaging data (**Figure 2**).

2.2 Surgical technique

The patient was placed in the operating room as for pterional craniotomy (**Figure 3**). Head rotation is carried out depending on the location of the aneurysm:

- 15° for ipsilateral Sylvian fissure, MCA aneurysms
- 20–30° for ICA
- 40–60° for Acom aneurysms

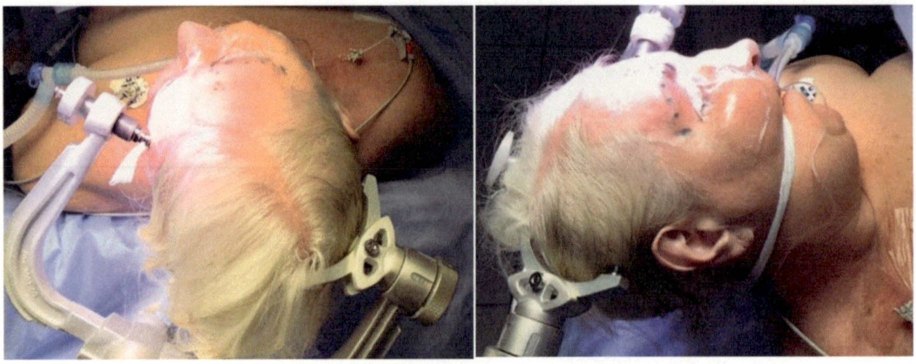

Figure 3.
Position of the patient on the operating table. The head is fixed in a Mayfield clamp, rotated to the contralateral side.

The zygomatic process is the highest point. This head position provides gravitational retraction of the frontal lobe away from the anterior cranial fossa to facilitate a subfrontal approach. The final position of both the head end and the entire operating table was determined intraoperatively after craniotomy and durotomy and can be changed by rotating the surgical table for better visualization.

2.3 Skin incision and soft tissue dissection

Primarily marked the skin above the eyebrow. The eyebrow was not shaved. For protection of the cornea and sclera, an aseptic ophthalmic gel was placed subconjunctivally. Before the start of the operation, the supraorbital notch was palpated, since it serves as the medial border of the skin incision.

The skin incision was made along the eyebrow, from the level of the supraorbital notch and further within the eyebrow, sometimes extending a few millimetres laterally beyond the hairline (**Figure 4**). The incision planning line is not linear, but somewhat curved (follows the line of the eyebrow) and runs in the mediolateral direction in relation to the hair follicles to avoid postoperative alopecia.

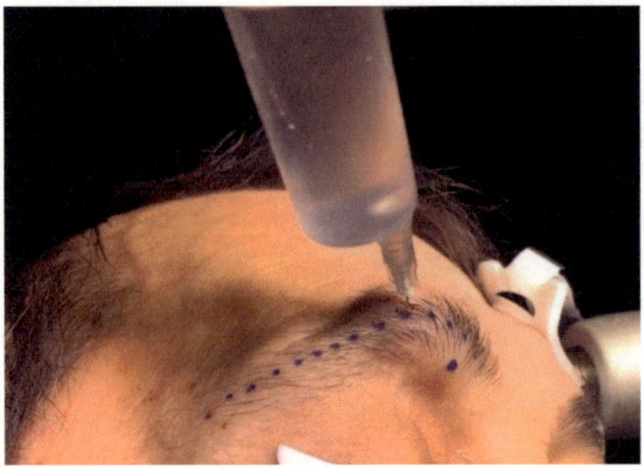

Figure 4.
Intraoperative photography. A - Marked skin incision along the eyebrow in ESA. B - the area of the planned incision is infiltrated with an anaesthetic with a vasoconstrictor (optional).

Initially, only the skin was incised. Next, layer-by-layer dissection of fat tissue and the frontalis muscle was performed. The supraorbital nerve and artery, the frontal branch of the facial nerve, and the superficial temporal artery were preserved.

The frontal muscle is cut parallel to the skin incision by monopolar coagulation and then the supraorbital region is skeletonized. The area of bone skeletonization must be at least 3 cm in diameter. The frontal muscle itself was stitched and retracted to the orbit.

After dissection of the frontalis muscle, additional skeletonization of the soft tissues was performed with a raspator, then the frontalis muscle was sutured and retracted to the orbit. Skin tensioners in the amount of three pieces were installed on the upper edge of the wound. The burr hole was placed with a high-speed drill (5 mm) at a key point just below the temporal line above the level of the base of the anterior cranial fossa. The direction of the craniotomy handle is important. To visualize the dura mater, it is necessary to resect with a burr parallel to the anterior cranial fossa, and not towards the orbit. After applying a single burr hole, dissection of the dura within the trefination and careful dissection along the periphery is necessary. To visualize the base of the anterior cranial fossa, as a rule, the inner plate of the bone was resected from the burr hole with a bur or pistol cutters.

The main task in craniotomy is to cut out a bone flap of the required size (at least 2–2.5 cm) with a minimum bone rim, preserve the dura mater, exclude penetration into the frontal sinus and damage to the supraorbital nerve. The first cut was made parallel to the upper edge of the orbit in the medial direction. The second cut was made upward and in a C-shape towards the medial point of the first cut (**Figures 5** and **6**).

If the examination reveals large frontal sinuses, it is necessary to plan osteotomy, avoiding penetration into the latter by lateralizing the approach or choosing an alternative craniotomy. Even though wide sinuses are not a contraindication, but they can increase the risk of cerebrospinal fluid (CSF) rhinorrhea and infectious complications. In some cases, the use of neuronavigation helps to avoid frontal sinus damage (**Figure 7**).

In the case of penetration into the frontal sinus, the tactics depend on the amount of penetration. With a small penetration without damaging the mucous membrane, it is sufficient to coat this area with wax. If the sinus mucosa is damaged, the latter is removed and coagulated, tamponated with muscle or fatty tissue with vancomycin,

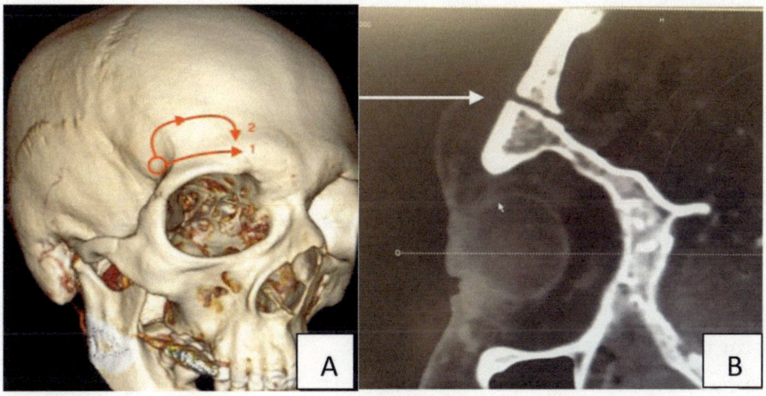

Figure 5.
Stages of planning the ESA. A - the sequence of cuts in ESA, B - the arrow shows the direction of the cut in the supraorbital region.

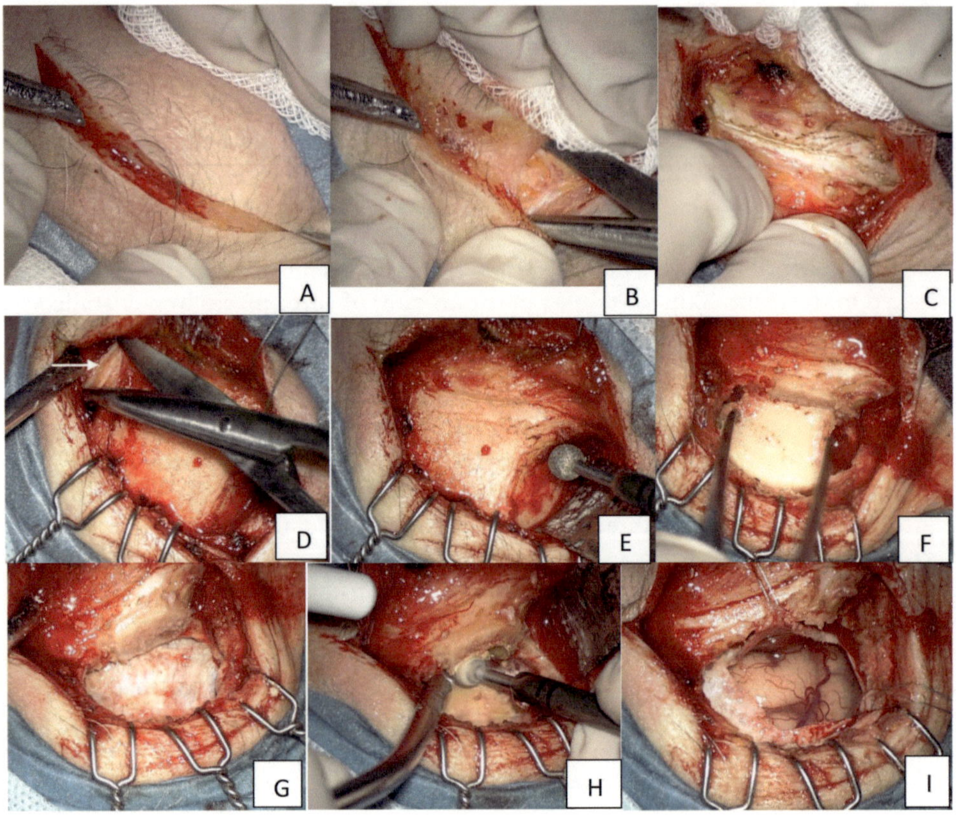

Figure 6.
A - incision along the eyebrow, B, C - dissection of soft tissues, transection of the frontalis muscle, D - identification of the supraorbital nerve (arrow), E - burr hole in the key point, F,G - view after osteotomy, H - resection of the supraorbital margin with a diamond burr, I – final view after durotomy.

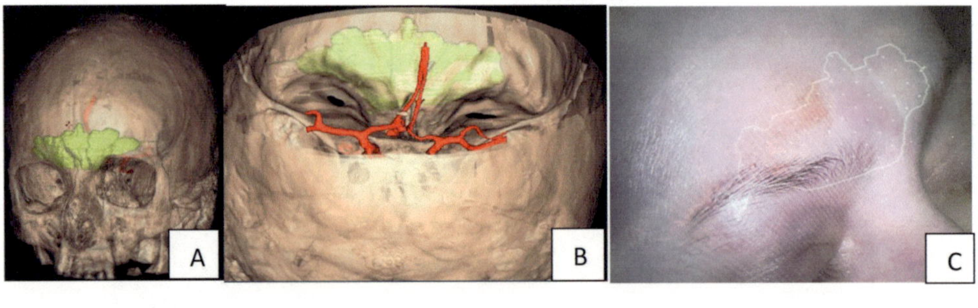

Figure 7.
The use of neuronavigation to assess the topography of the frontal sinus. A, B – 3D model shows the topography of the frontal sinuses, C - through a microscope, the boundaries of the frontal sinuses are visualized.

and then closed with a periosteal flap. Hermetic closure of the dura mater is extremely important for the prevention of complications.

The bone flap is placed in place and fixed with miniplates (**Figure 8**).

The temporal fascia and muscle were sutured to the periosteum. The subcutaneous tissue and skin were sutured in layers using 4–0 or 5–0 Prolene. Postoperative drainage was not used.

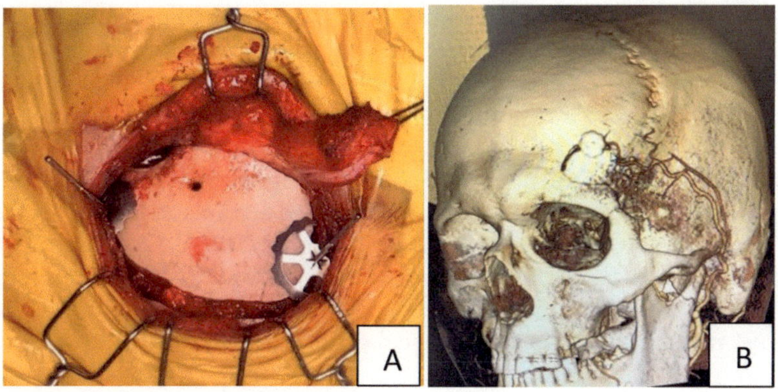

Figure 8.
Clinical example of bone flap fixation. A – intraoperative view after fixation with craniofixes, B – postoperative CT scan with reconstruction.

2.4 Postoperative management

The early postoperative period includes the management of the patient in the conditions of the neurocritical care unit, usually within 12–24 hours after the intervention. The patient and staff are warned about the possibility of developing periorbital

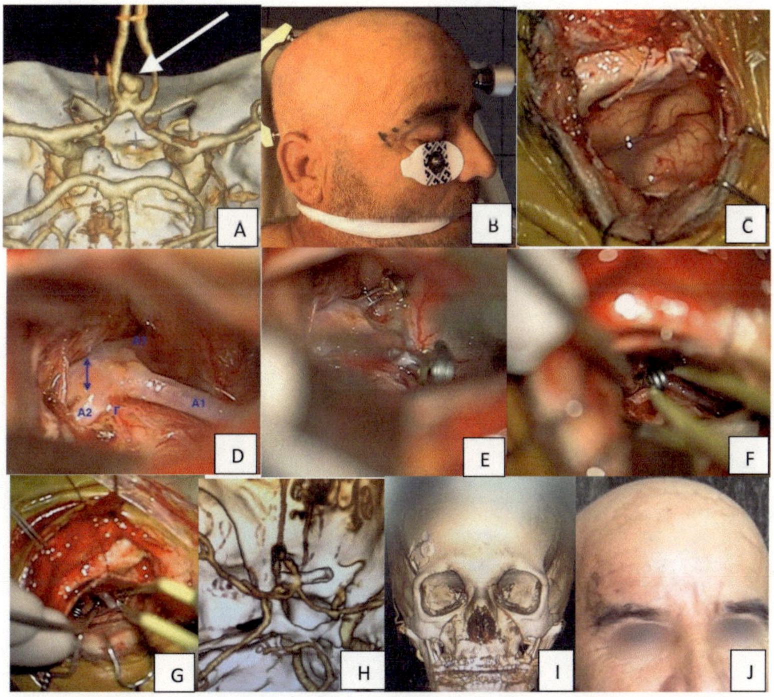

Figure 9.
Clinical case. A – CT Angio – AcomA aneurysm, B – marking of the eyebrow incision, C – intraoperative view after opening the dura mater, D – intraoperative view after dissection of the ACA-AcomA complex, A1 – A2 segments of the ACA, A2 – A2 segment of the ACA, arrow marks the aneurysm neck, E – temporary clipping of A1 segments of the ACA from both sides, F – clipping of the aneurysm neck, G – view before suturing the dura mater, H – postoperative CT angiography, I – craniography with reconstruction, J-view patient one month after surgery.

oedema, which we observed in all patients. For the purpose of prevention, it is necessary to use ice locally within 1 hour after the operation. Periorbital oedema may persist during the first 2–5 days after the intervention and lead to transient brow ptosis.

We present clinical observations of the use of ESA in different locations of aneurysms.

Clinical example of Acom aneurysm clipping (**Figure 9**).

Man 54 years old. Debut of the disease with a sudden severe headache. Suffering from hypertension, with a rise in blood pressure up to 200/100 mmHg. CT scan of the brain revealed no data for subarachnoid haemorrhage (SAH). CT angiography revealed a saccular aneurysm in the upper PSA region. In the neurological status there are headache, nausea, and severe meningeal syndrome. No focal neurological disorders were identified (**Figure 9**).

Clinical example of Pcom aneurysm clipping (**Figure 10**).

A 75-year-old woman. Onset of the disease with a severe headache, mainly in the occipital region, vomiting. In the neurological status, headache and severe meningeal syndrome. No focal signs.

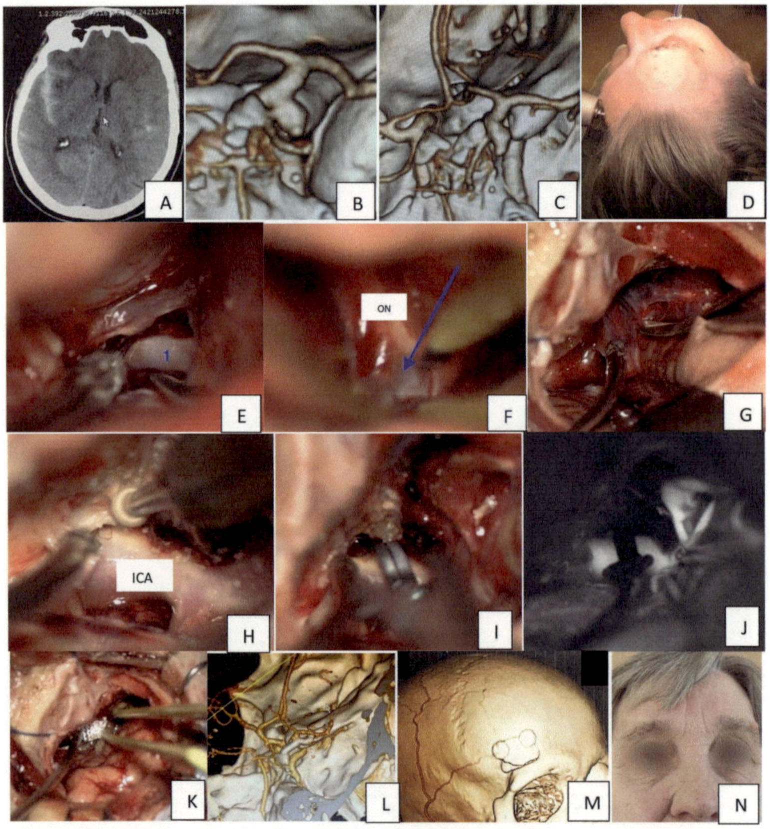

Figure 10.
Clinical example A – CT scan, SAH is visualized in the right Sylvian fissure, B, C – ICA aneurysm at the orifice of the Pcom, D – positioning of the patient with head rotation, E – intraoperative view, the ICA is visualized (1) and blood clots in carotid cistern, E – intraoperative view, arrow shows terminal membrane of the third ventricle and optic nerve (ON), G – dissection of the Sylvian fissure, H – intradural resection of the anterior clinoid process, I – stage of aneurysm clipping, J – intraoperative angiography with indocyanine green, K – view before closure of the DM, L, M – CT angiography and craniography with reconstruction, N – view of the patient 4 weeks after the operation.

3. Minipterional approach

Minipterional approach (MPA) is a limited model of pterional approach, the centre of which is the Sylvian fissure [11–13]. Therefore, the main indications for MPA are patients with MCA and ICA aneurysms. MPA can be an alternative to minimally invasive anterolateral approaches for patients with large frontal sinuses.

3.1 Anatomical access landmarks

Pterion is one of the key landmarks of the MPA and the area of the burr hole placement (**Figure 11**). It is localized in the region of the temporal fossa and is a point at the junction of the parietal bone, the squamous part of the temporal bone, the greater wing of the sphenoid bone and the frontal bone. These bones in the region of the pterion are connected with a sphenoparietal, coronary and squamous suture. Immediately below the pterion, the anterior Sylvian point is located. This landmark is the most common for entry and further dissection of the Sylvian fissure, since the cistern of the Sylvian fissure is usually dilated in this area.

3.2 Surgical technique

The patient is positioned like for pterional approach. An arcuate incision of the skin and soft tissues of 4–5 cm was performed within the scalp. In the temporal region, the incision was started 1–1.5 cm above the zygomatic process and anteriorly from the superficial temporal artery and continued anteriorly to the projection of the superior temporal line (**Figure 12**).

The incision of the superficial fascia and temporalis muscle was carried out in a C-shaped manner with the base towards the pterion. After subperiosteal dissection, the temporalis muscle was brought together using hook tensioners. This allows the pterion area to be completely exposed. The burr hole was placed upwards from the

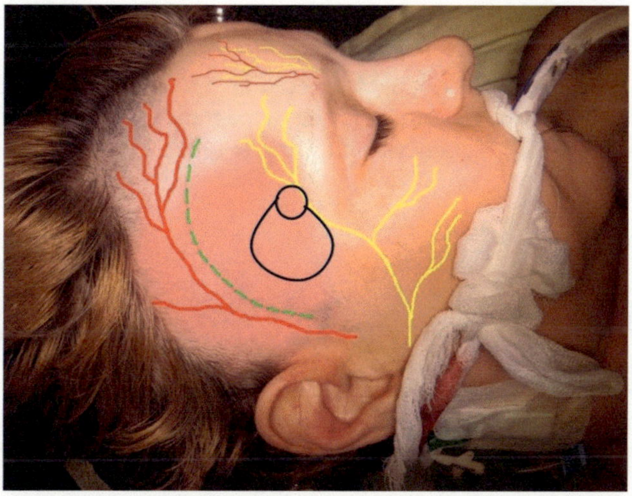

Figure 11.
Intraoperative photography. Schematic representation of the main anatomical landmarks of MPA. Bone borders are marked in black. Skin incision marked in green. Arrows: white - supraorbital nerve and artery, red - branches of the frontal branch of the facial nerve, blue - superficial temporal artery.

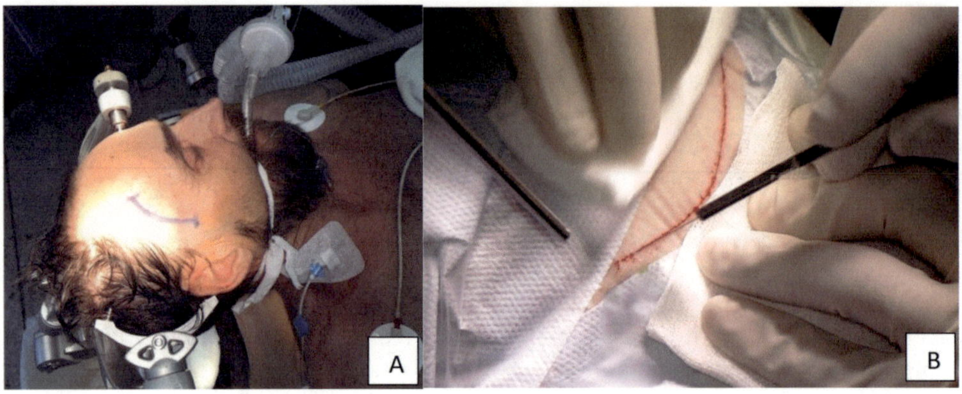

Figure 12.
Intraoperative photography. A, B - Skin incision marked for MPA.

fronto-zygomatic suture immediately below the superior temporal line. A 2–3 cm craniotomy includes the lateral portions of the sphenoid bone, part of the frontal bone below the superior temporal line, and a minimal portion of the temporal bone. As in the case of classical pterional approach, the crest of the sphenoid bone was resected with cutters and a bur until the meningoorbital artery was visualized in the superior orbital fissure (**Figure 13**).

The durotomy was performed with a semi-oval incision with the base towards the pterion. After opening the dura mater, the Sylvian fissure was visualized in the centre of the wound, which indicates the correct location of the craniotomy. The intradural stage of surgery was performed under microscopic magnification using traditional microneurosurgical techniques.

After clipping of the aneurysm and verification of its complete exclusion, hemostasis was performed. The dura mater was sutured hermetically. In order to prevent pneumocephalus, the subdural space was irrigated with saline until a distinct brain pulsation appeared and air was forced out. The bone flap was fixed with craniofixes or miniplates. The temporal fascia/muscle, subcutaneous tissue, and skin were sutured in layers (**Figure 14**).

Subcutaneous drainage was not performed due to the small size of craniotomy. Postoperative management is identical to the management of patients after ESA.

Clinical example of MCA aneurysm clipping (**Figure 15**).

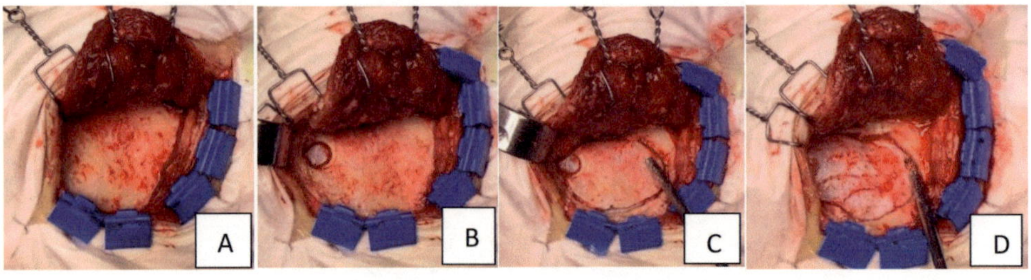

Figure 13.
Intraoperative photos, MPA on the right. A – intraoperative view, skin-aponeurotic flap and temporal muscle are reduced anteriorly, B – burr hole is placed in the area of the pterion, C – bone flap is sawn out, D – view after craniotomy.

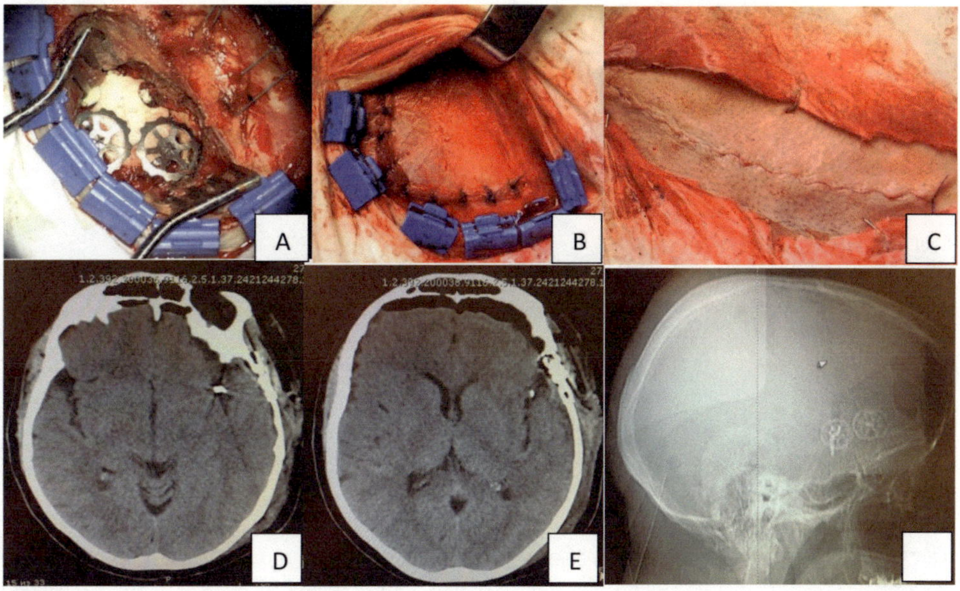

Figure 14.
Intraoperative photographs. A - the bone flap is put in place and fixed, B,C - sutures on the temporal muscle and skin, D,E,F - CT and craniography.

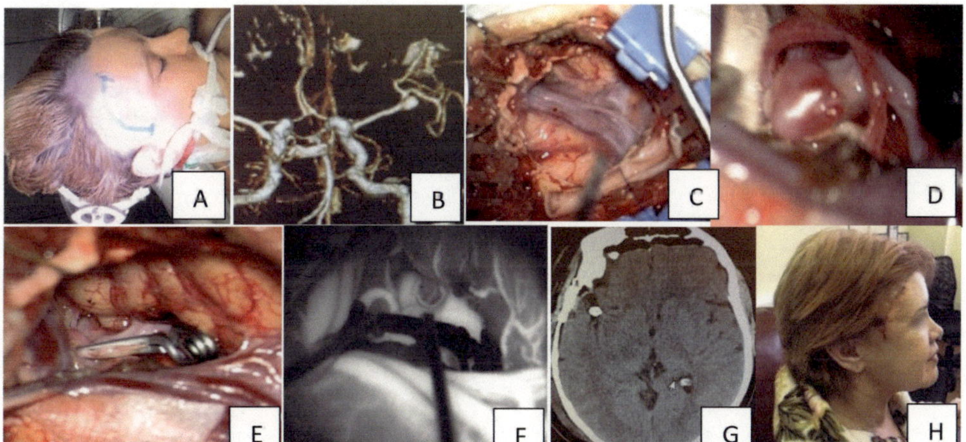

Figure 15.
A - marking of the planned incision, B - CT angiography - saccular aneurysm M1 of the segment of the MCA on the left, C - intraoperative view after minipterional craniotomy and opening of the dura, the centre of craniotomy over the Sylvian fissure, D - saccular aneurysm M1 of the segment of the MCA, E - clipping of the aneurysm, F – intraoperative angiography with indocyanine green, aneurysm is excluded from the cerebral circulation, MCA branches are visualized, G – craniography and CT after surgery, H – view of the patient a week after surgery.

A 62-year-old woman with unruptured MCA aneurysm.

Clinical example of ophthalmic aneurysm clipping (**Figure 16**).

A 30-year-old woman with unruptured ophthalmic artery aneurysm.

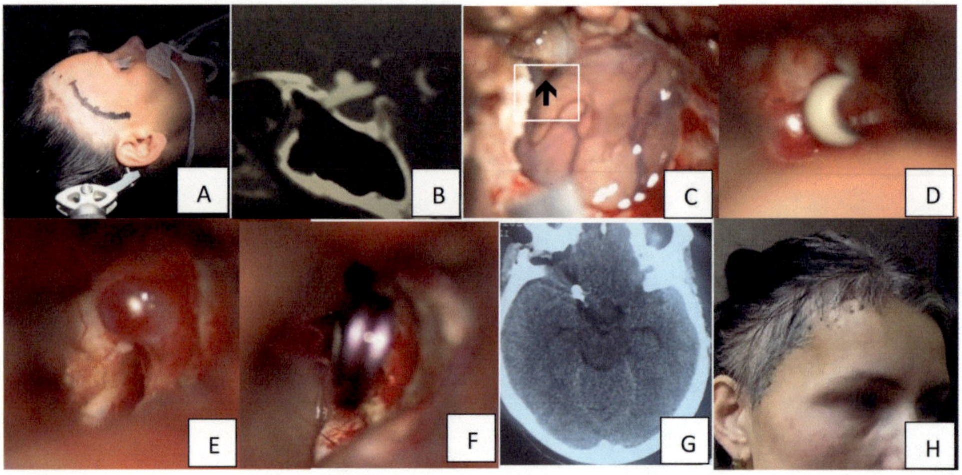

Figure 16.
A - marking of the planned incision, B - CT angiography - carotid-ophthalmic aneurysm is visualized on the right, C - intraoperative view after MPA and opening of the dura, the Sylvian fissure is marked with an arrow, D - intradural resection of the ACP with a 2-mm diamond burr E – aneurysm lateral to the optic nerve, F –clipping of the aneurysm, G – postoperative CT, H – view of the patient 2 weeks after surgery.

4. Transorbital approaches

Transorbital approaches, due to the inclusion of the upper wall of the orbit in the bone flap, increase the free space for working with microinstruments, significantly reduce the distance to the target of surgery, and reduce brain retraction. This made it possible to expand indications in aneurysm surgery, for example, to use this approach for large and giant aneurysms, small unruptured basilar aneurysms. The main modifications of transorbital approaches include:

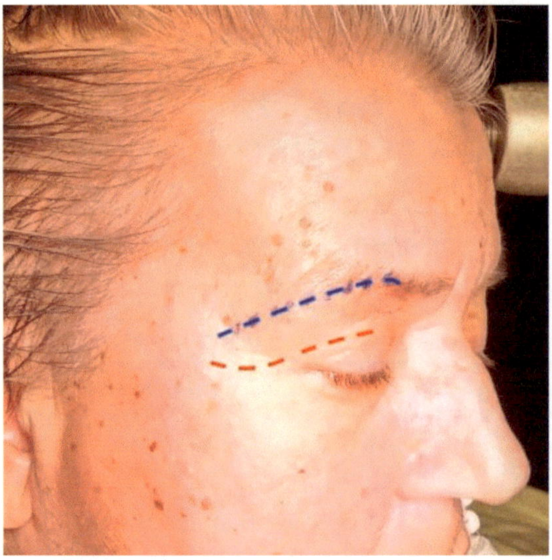

Figure 17.
Various types of skin incisions for transorbital craniotomy. A - eyebrow (blue), B - transpalpebral (red).

1. Eyebrow transorbital approach (ETA)

2. Transpalpebral transorbital approach (TPTA)

Despite different types of skin incisions, the stage of osteotomy is identical, but the functional and cosmetic outcomes are significantly different (**Figure 17**).

4.1 Eyebrow transorbital approach

The skin incision was made along the eyebrow in accordance with the described guidelines for ESA. The planning of transorbital approach is identical to ESA and requires a thorough assessment of the topography of the frontal sinuses [14, 15]. With a high risk of penetration of the frontal sinus, the choice of lateralization of the bone window or the choice of a traditional approach will be correct.

Indications for ETA:

- Aneurysms of the anterior circulation: ICA, Acom, A1 segment of ACA, MCA of M1-M2 segments, excluding distal ones.

- Small unruptured upper basilar artery aneurysm

- Anatomical access landmarks are shown in **Figure 18**.

4.1.1 Surgical technique

Patient positioning and head rotation are identical to those for pterional craniotomy and depends on aneurysm location. For all transorbital approaches, a temporary tarsorrhaphy was necessarily performed with preliminary placement

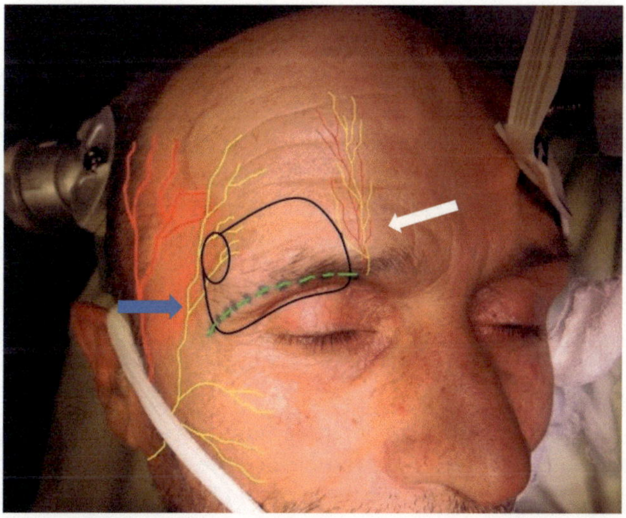

Figure 18.
Intraoperative photo. Schematic representation of the main anatomical landmarks of access. Bone borders are marked in black. The skin incision is marked in green. Branches of the superficial temporal artery are marked in red. Arrows: white - supraorbital nerve and artery, blue - frontal branch of the facial nerve.

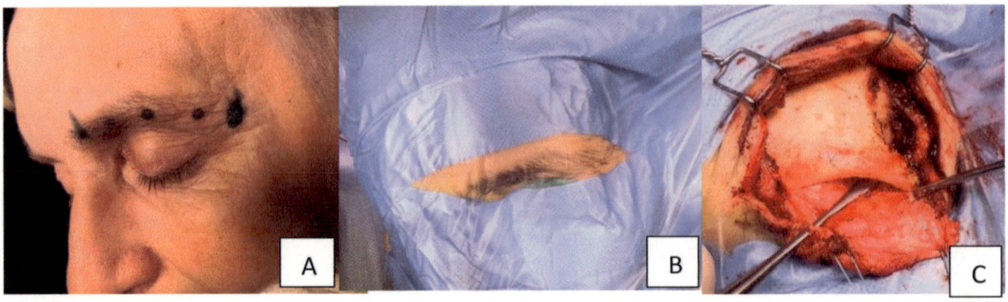

Figure 19.
Intraoperative view, A, B – soft tissue incision along the eyebrow, C – subperiosteal dissection of the supraorbital region of the frontal bone, the edge of the orbit and the zygomatic process of the frontal bone.

of an antiseptic gel subconjunctivally. A skin incision was made directly along the eyebrow, starting from the level of the pupillary line and continuing laterally within the eyebrow, sometimes extending several millimetres laterally. The supraorbital nerve and artery, the frontal branch of the facial nerve, and the superficial temporal artery are always preserved. The initial stage of incision and dissection of the frontalis muscle is identical to that in ESA, however, after transection of the frontalis muscle, careful skeletonization of the upper edge of the orbit was performed from the level of the supraorbital foramen to the fronto-zygomatic suture. Dissection of the contents of the orbit lateral to the fronto-zygomatic suture should be avoided due to the risk of damage to the lateral canthal ligament and impaired movement of the upper eyelid with the formation of a temporary or permanent diastasis when the eyelids is closed. During dissection, special attention was paid to the preservation of the periosteum and periorbital tissue. The temporal muscle was separated from its place of attachment at the level of the superior temporal line and brought down with a retractor towards the temporal fossa (**Figure 19**).

A single burr hole was made downward from the temporal line immediately above the level of the base of the anterior cranial fossa, at the key point. The trans-orbital approach included the roof of the orbit, a portion of the frontal bone, and approximately 1–1.5 cm of the zygomatic bone. A single bone flap was sawn out using a craniotome and a high-speed burr. The diameter of the bone window is approximately 25–30 mm. The first cut was made from the burr hole upwards in the supraorbital region, describing a C-shaped bend towards the upper wall of the orbit. From the side of the orbit, the contents of which are protected with a spatula, a cut was also made using a craniotome towards the line of the previous cut. In the area of the zygomatic process, sawing towards the key point can be carried out both with a craniotome and with an oscillating saw, using the protection of the contents of the orbit with a spatula. The roof of the orbit was broken using a chisel. After osteotomy, sharp edges were resected in the area of the upper wall of the orbit with a bur and wire cutters (**Figure 20**).

If necessary, extradural resection of the sphenoid bone and anterior clinoid process performed the degree of bony resection depends on the location and size of the aneurysm. All manipulations were performed through minimal craniotomy. Upon completion of the necessary resection of the bone structures, the dura mater was opened with a semi-oval incision with the base towards the orbit. Then, the surgical technique is dictated by the location and size of the aneurysm.

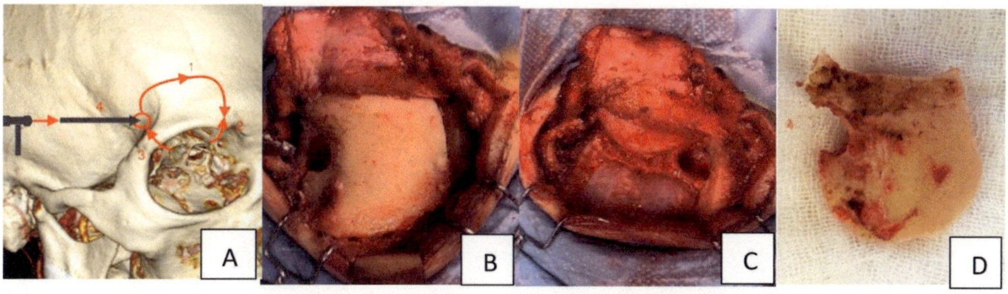

Figure 20.
Planning and stages of ETA. A – the sequence of cuts (the arrow indicates the key hole from which the upper wall of the orbit is broken with a chisel), B – the burr hole is placed at the key point and the bone is cut away from the supraorbital hole towards the key point, C – view of the bone flap, D – performed transorbital access, frontal sinus opened.

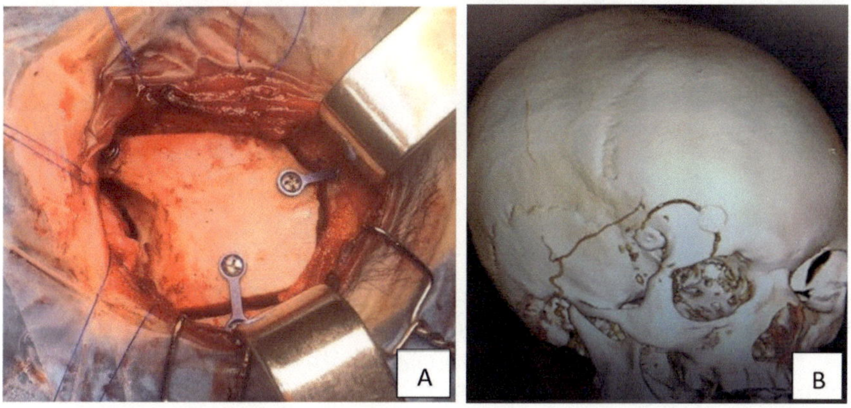

Figure 21.
Intraoperative view. A - The bone flap is put in place and fixed with miniplates. B – CT craniography after minitransorbital craniotomy.

Classical microsurgical technique is used. Wound closure is standard and has been described above (**Figure 21**).

4.2 Transpalpebral transorbital approach

The transpalpebral approach, or access through the upper eyelid, is borrowed from ophthalmic and plastic surgery. Transpalpebral approach has been used in neurosurgical practice since 2008 and includes an incision along the natural crease of the upper eyelid followed by a minimal fronto-orbital craniotomy [16–18]. In fact, the TPTA trajectory is identical to the ESA and ETA and provides access to the anterior cranial fossa, the parasellar space.

The indications for TPTA are identical to those for ETA.

4.2.1 Anatomical access landmarks

Knowledge of anatomy is an indispensable condition for ensuring the effectiveness and safety of surgical intervention. Anatomical landmarks are similar to ETA (**Figure 22**).

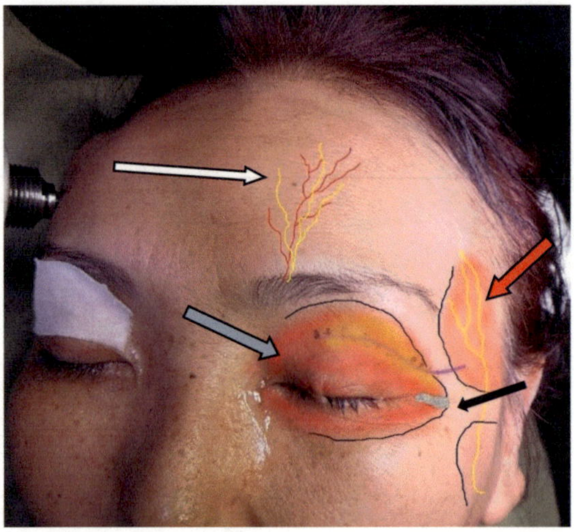

Figure 22.
Intraoperative view. Schematic representation of the main anatomical landmarks of access. Bone borders are marked in black. Arrows: white - supraorbital nerve and artery, grey - circular muscle of the eye, black - lateral cantal ligament, red - temporalis muscle with branches of the frontal branch of the facial nerve.

4.2.2 Surgical technique

The eyebrow and eyelid area are prepped with antiseptic solutions, an ophthalmic gel was applied subconjunctivally. Next, a temporary tarsorrhaphy was performed with a 5–0 thread. The planned incision area was infiltrated with an anaesthetic solution and a vasoconstrictor. The incision was made along the natural fold of the upper eyelid from the level of the supraorbital opening 3.5–4 cm long. If necessary, the incision can be extended laterally by several millimetres exclusively within the fold. The incision should start at least 10 mm above the upper edge of the eyelid and at least 5–6 mm above the projection of the lateral canthal ligament. Thus, the incision is planned below the supraorbital and frontotemporal branches of the facial nerve, which makes it possible to exclude negative cosmetic consequences associated with nerve damage. Initially, the incision was made through the skin and the orbicular muscle of the eye while maintaining the orbital septum. Damage to the orbicularis muscle must be minimized as the blood supply to the eyelid passes through the orbicularis muscle. A single musculoskeletal flap was formed, which ensures adequate healing. Dissection by the sharp way was carried out mainly in the upper and lateral direction. At this stage, the upper and lateral edges of the orbit were palpated for control. Next, a subperiosteal dissection of the supraorbital region, the upper lateral edge of the orbit, and the zygomatic process of the frontal bone was performed with visualization of the fronto-zygomatic suture. During dissection, special attention was paid to the preservation of the periosteum and periorbital tissue. The temporalis muscle was dissected by monopolar coagulation from the place of its attachment at the level of the superior temporal line. Limitation of muscle dissection, its dissection and devascularization eliminates the formation of a depression in this area.

A minimal orbitofrontal craniotomy included the roof of the orbit, a portion of the frontal bone, and approximately 1–1.5 cm of the frontal process of the zygomatic bone. A single bone flap was sawn out using a craniotome and a high-speed burr. The diameter of the bone defect was no more than 25–30 mm. After

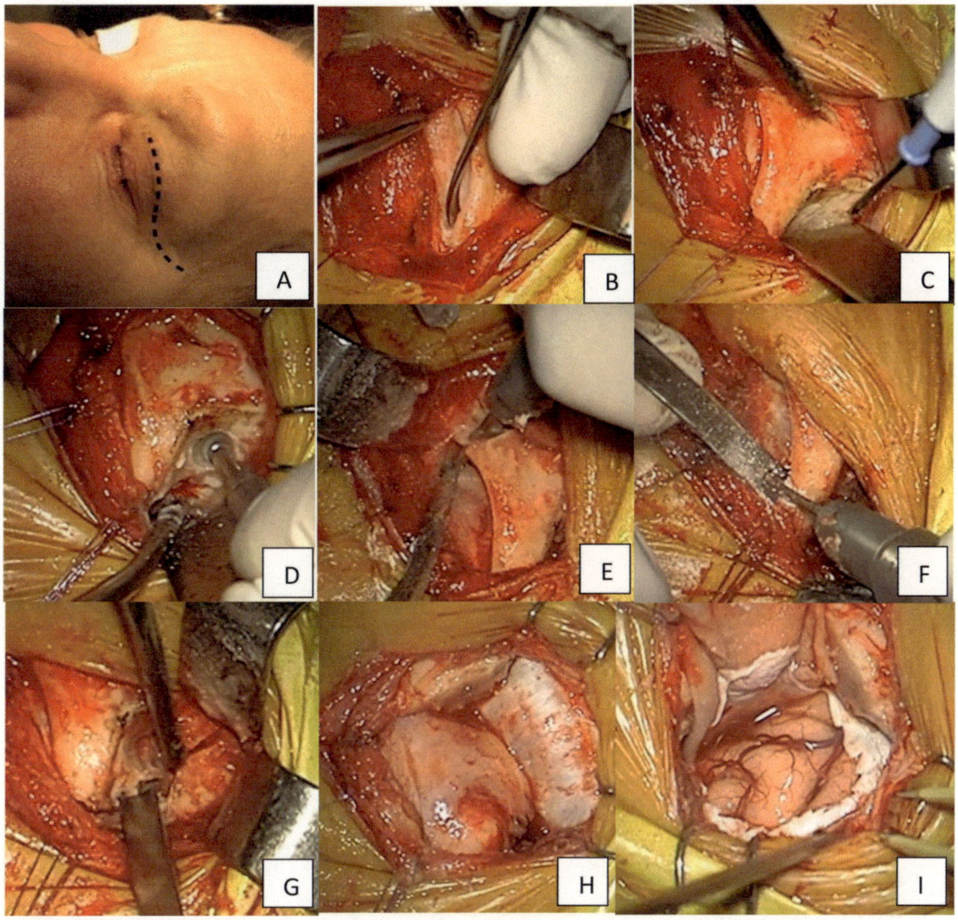

Figure 23.
Intraoperative view, A – soft tissue incision along the natural crease of the upper eyelid, B – mobilization of the upper wall of the orbit, C – dissection of a part of the temporal muscle over the area of application of the burr hole, D – burr hole is applied at a key point, E – propyl in the area of the frontal process of the zygomatic bones, above the fronto-zygomatic suture. E – cut in the region of the upper wall of the orbit, medial to the supraorbital notch, G – using a chisel, the upper wall of the orbit is broken, H – view after craniotomy, I – the dura mater is opened with the base to the orbit.

craniotomy, the roof of the orbit was broken using a chisel. If necessary, extradural resection of the anterior clinoid process and decompression of the optic nerve canal were performed from this access. When opening the frontal sinus, the defect was closed according to the previously described principles. The dura mater was opened with a semi-oval incision with the base towards the orbit. Additionally, tension sutures were placed on the edges of the dura mater to increase the viewing angle and epidural hemostasis (**Figure 23**).

At the end of the intervention, the bone flap was fixed with miniplates. The wound was sutured in three layers: muscle, subcutaneous tissue and skin. The temporalis muscle can be fixed to miniplates or to holes formed in the area of the upper lateral wall of the orbit. The orbicular muscle of the eye was sutured with a 4–0 absorbable suture. An intradermal suture was applied using a 5–0 or 6–0 suture. Postoperative drainage was not used.

Clinical example of ophthalmic aneurysm clipping through ETA (**Figure 24**).

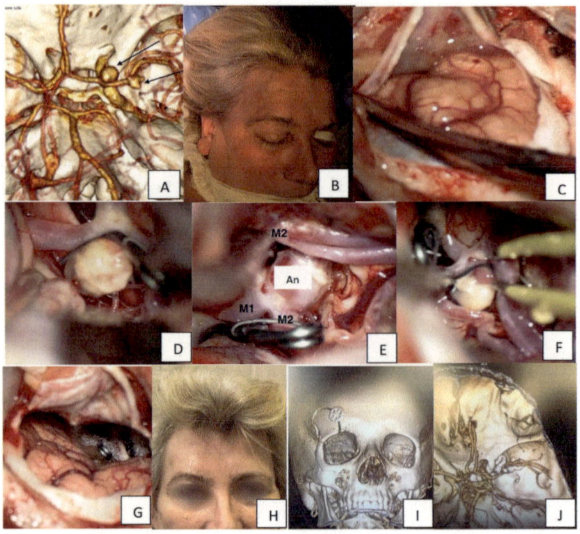

Figure 24.
Clinical example of clipping of multiple ETA aneurysms. A –CT angiography, B- intraoperative view, position of the patient on the table, incision marking; C – view after opening the dura mater; D – intraoperative view after dissection and clipping of the ICA bifurcation aneurysm; ICA, E – dissection of the aneurysm (An) of the MCA bifurcation with visualization of the M1 and M2 branches of the MCA, G – view after clipping of the aneurysm, H – view of the patient 1 month after surgery, I, J – postoperative CT craniography with reconstruction, CT angiography.

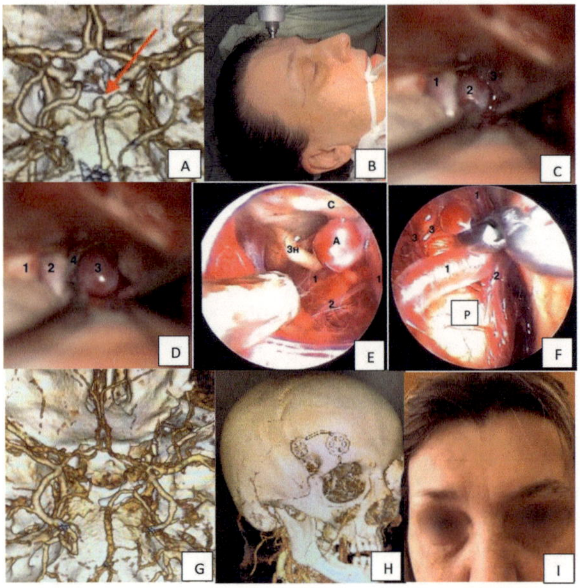

Figure 25.
Clinical example. A – CT angiography, basilar artery aneurysm, B – Intraoperative view of planning a skin incision along the natural fold of the upper eyelid on the right, C – intraoperative view through the retrocarotid space: 1 – ICA, 2 – aneurysm, 3 – PCA P1 segment, D – view through the retrocarotid space: 1 – optic nerve, 2 - ICA, 3 - Aneurysm, 4 – posterior cerebral artery (PCA), P1 segment on the left, E - view through the endoscope 0°: 1 - PCA, 2 - Pecheron artery, C - clivus, 3n - oculomotor nerve, A - aneurysm, E – view through the 0° endoscope. After clipping: 1 - PCA, 2 – superior cerebellar artery, 3 - Pecheron artery, P - pons, G - control of CT angiography - a clip is visualized. H - during bone reconstruction, the volume of the craniotomy is visualized, I - is the view of the patient after 2 months.

A 58-year-old woman with multiple unruptured aneurysm: ICA terminus and MCA artery aneurysms.

Clinical example of basilar bifurcation aneurysm clipping through TPTA (**Figure 25**).

A 53-year-old woman unruptured basilar bifurcation artery aneurysm.

5. Conclusion

In summary, it should be noted that the surgical approach is an important stage of the entire intervention, which can determine the outcomes of patients. Today, highly informative neuroimaging, coupled with modern neurosurgical microscopes, endoscopy and microinstrumentation, substantiate a completely different approach to the surgical treatment of cerebral aneurysms, an approach that is based on individual anatomy: facial, bone, and vascular. An approach that provides a choice between a traditional approach, a minimally invasive approach, or the use of the endovascular intervention. The main task of a neurosurgeon is the correct choice of treatment method depending on the individual neuroimaging pattern and the patient's condition. The main goal of individualization is to create the shortest efficient route to the target with minimal collateral damage, ensuring the safety of the intervention. Sufficient experience in microsurgical aneurysm clipping and proper selection of patients allows us to use different minimally invasive approaches safely and effectively.

Conflict of interest

The authors declare no conflict of interest.

Consent of patients

All of patients gave their consent to the publication of their photos in this article.

Author details

Revaz Dzhindzhikhadze[1,2], Renat Kambiev[2], Andrey Polyakov[2]*, Andrey Zaitsev[2], Anton Ermolaev[2] and Igor Bogdanovich[2]

1 Russian Medical Academy of Continuous Professional Education, Moscow, Russia

2 Moscow Regional Research and Clinical Institute ("MONIKI"), Moscow, Russia

*Address all correspondence to: ap.neurosurg@mail.ru

References

[1] Yasargil MG, Fox JL, Ray MW. The operative approach to aneurysms of the anterior communicating artery. In: Krayenbühl H, editor. Advances and Technical Standards in Neurosurgery. Vol. 2. Vienna: Springer Verlag; 1975. pp. 113-170. DOI: 10.1007/978-3-7091-7088-5

[2] Mohale DG, Naicker D, Ndlovu B, Leola K, Dlamini M, Gardner B, et al. Keyhole approaches applied to clipping of acutely ruptured intracerebral Aneurysms-A technical note and case series. World Neurosurgery. 2022;**168**:209-218. DOI: 10.1016/j.wneu.2022.10.029 Epub 2022 Oct 13

[3] Mori K, Watanabe S. Keyhole approach in cerebral aneurysm surgeries. Advances and Technical Standards in Neurosurgery. 2022;**44**:265-275. DOI: 10.1007/978-3-030-87649-4_15

[4] Prajapati H, Ansari A, Jaiswal M. Keyhole approach in anterior circulation aneurysm: Current indication, advantages, technical limitations, complications and their avoidance. Journal of Cerebrovascular and Endovascular Neurosurgery. 2022;**24**(2):101-112. DOI: 10.7461/jcen.2022.E2021.07.008

[5] Reisch R, Perneczky A, Filippi R. Surgical technique of the supraorbital keyhole craniotomy. Surgical Neurology. 2003;**59**:223-227. DOI: 10.1016/s0090-3019(02)01037-6

[6] Reisch R, Perneczky A. Ten-year experience with the supraorbital subfrontal approach through an eyebrow skin incision. Neurosurgery. 2005;**57**(4 Suppl):242-255. DOI: 10.1227/01.neu.0000178353.42777.2c

[7] Rychen J, Croci D, Roethlisberger M, Nossek E, Potts MB, Radovanovic I, et al. Keyhole approaches for surgical treatment of intracranial aneurysms: A short review. Neurological Research. 2019;**41**(1):68-76. DOI: 10.1080/01616412.2018.1531202

[8] Bhatoe HS. Supraorbital keyhole approach for clipping ruptured anterior circulation aneurysms. Neurology India. 2020;**68**(5):1028-1029. DOI: 10.4103/0028-3886.294829

[9] Ong V, Faung B, Brown NJ, Yang C, Sahyouni R, Ng E, et al. Supraorbital keyhole craniotomy for clipping cerebral aneurysms: A systematic review and meta-analysis. World Neurosurgery. 2022;**168**:287-297.e1. DOI: 10.1016/j.wneu.2022.09.129

[10] Van Lindert E, Perneczky A, Fries G, Pierangeli E. The supraorbital keyhole approach to supratentorial aneurysms: Concept and technique. Surgical Neurology. 1998;**49**:481-490. DOI: 10.1016/s0090-3019(96)00539-3

[11] Di Bonaventura R, Sturiale CL, Latour K, Mazzucchi E, Marchese E, Albanese A. Comparison between Minipterional craniotomy associated with focused sylvian fissure opening and standard Pterional approach with extended sylvian fissure dissection for treatment of unruptured middle cerebral artery aneurysms. World Neurosurgery. 2021;**146**:e1293-e1300. DOI: 10.1016/j.wneu.2020.11.150

[12] Martinez-Perez R, Tsimpas A, Joswig H, Hernandez-Alvarez V, Mura J. Extradural minipterional approach for giant intracranial aneurysms. Surgical Neurology International. 2020;**11**:382. DOI: 10.25259/SNI_368_2020

[13] Rychen J, Saemann A, Gehweiler JE, Roethlisberger M, Soleman J, Hutter G,

et al. The sylvian keyhole approach for surgical clipping of middle cerebral artery aneurysms: Technical nuance to the minipterional craniotomy. Frontiers in Surgery. 2022;**9**:1078735. DOI: 10.3389/fsurg.2022.1078735

[14] Dare A, Landi M, Lopes D, Grand W. Eyebrow incision for combined orbital osteotomy and supraorbital minicraniotomy: Application to aneurysms of the anterior circulation. Journal of Neurosurgery. 2001;**95**:714-718. DOI: 10.3171/jns.2001.95.4.0714

[15] Lee Warren W, Grant G. Transciliary orbitofrontozygomatic approach to the lesions of the anterior cranial fossa. Neurosurgery. 2009;**64**(Suppl. 2):ons324-ons330. DOI: 10.1227/01.NEU.0000338951.29171.07

[16] Abdel Aziz K, Bhatia S, Tantawy M, Sekula R, Keller J, Froelich S, et al. Minimally invasive transpalpebral "eyelid" approach to the anterior cranial base. Neurosurgery. 2011;**69**(2 Suppl Operative):ons195-ons206. DOI: 10.1227/NEU.0b013e31821c3ea3

[17] Dzhindzhikhadze RS, Dreval ON, Lazarev VA, Polyakov AV. Transpalpebral approach in skull base surgery: How I do it. Acta Neurochirurgica. 2019;**161**:133-137. DOI: 10.1007/s00701-018-3724-4

[18] Dzhindzhikhadze R, Polyakov A, Kambiev R, et al. Transpalpebral approach for microsurgical clipping of an unruptured basilar apex aneurysm: Case report and literature review. British Journal of Neurosurgery. 2020;**30**:1-5. DOI: 10.1080/02688697.2020.1849543

Chapter 6

Clipping Strategies and Intraoperative Tools to Detect Aneurysm Obliteration and Cerebral Vessel Patency

Pasquale Anania and Pietro Fiaschi

Abstract

Cerebral aneurysms are common cerebrovascular diseases most frequently manifest with vascular rupture and subsequent subarachnoid hemorrhage. Microsurgical clipping is considered the best long-term treatment, despite of the increase of endovascular interventional treatments in the latest years. Vascular control is a pivotal concept for aneurysms surgery, which provides the application of temporary clip in case of rupture, whereas the application of permanent clip requires the perfect knowledge of aneurysm anatomy. Several techniques to obtain the obliteration of the aneurysm while preserving the parent vessels and its branches have been described. Micro-Doppler ultrasonography (MUSG), indocyanine green video angiography (ICG-VA), and electrophysiological neuromonitoring (IONM) are all useful intraoperative tools, which can improve the safety of surgical procedures and achieve the goal of aneurysm obliteration with parent vessel and perforating preservation.

Keywords: cerebral aneurysm, clipping techniques, indocyanine, micro-doppler, neuromonitoring

1. Introduction

Cerebral aneurysms are common cerebrovascular diseases with an incidence rate ranging between 2% and 6% [1, 2]. Aneurysm rupture is the most frequent presentation of intracranial aneurysm, causing intracranial hemorrhage, usually subarachnoid hemorrhage (SAH) [3, 4]. The incidence rate of SAH is about 6 to 8 cases per 100,000 in the western population, with about 10,000–20,000 cases per year [3]. SAH-associated mortality is 50% at 30 days, and only up to 30% of patients can return to normal life after SAH [3]. In the latest years, endovascular interventional treatments of intracranial aneurysms have increased rapidly, but microsurgical clipping is still considered the best long-term treatment for this disease [5–10].

Temporary blockage of the feeding artery of the aneurysm, associated with simple or multiple applications of clips along the neck, are techniques that can allow the dissection and remodeling of the neck with obliteration of the aneurysm [11, 12].

However, all these techniques are associated with the risk of parent vessel stenosis and perforating artery damage, leading to brain ischemic damage and neurological defect [1]. The morbidity related to ischemic complications of the surgery of cerebral aneurysms is up to 7.6% [13, 14]. Therefore, the goal of surgical treatment is an optimal obliteration of the aneurysms without residual, while preserving the parent vessels and their branches [5].

Micro-Doppler ultrasonography (MUSG), indocyanine green video angiography (ICG-VA), and electrophysiological neuromonitoring (IONM) are useful intraoperative tools that are used to improve the safety of surgical procedures and achieve the goal of aneurysm obliteration with parent vessel and perforating preservation [1, 5, 11].

The aim of this chapter is to describe the strategies for surgical treatment of cerebral aneurysms and the tools to detect the correct aneurysm obliteration and the patency of the parent vessel and its branches. These techniques allow for improving the safety of surgical procedures, while reducing the risk of aneurysm remnants and avoiding irreversible damage to the brain tissue with consequent neurological derangement.

2. Techniques of clipping

Despite the technical skills and expertise of the surgeon revest a pivotal role, aneurysms surgery is often associated with a high risk of intraoperative rupture because of the fragility of the aneurysm and surgical manipulation. For this reason, vascular control is a pivotal concept that the neurosurgeon must respect during aneurysms surgery. Vascular control means the exposition of the afferent and efferent arteries, which move blood to the aneurysm in anterograde and retrograde direction, respectively. Vascular control is mandatory to allow the application of temporary clip on the afferent artery and eventually on efferent arteries in case of difficult aneurysm dissection or intraoperative rupture. Permanent clipping means the application of a definitive clip on the neck of the aneurysm to arrest the blood flow into the dome [12].

2.1 Temporary clipping

Temporary clipping is the application of the clip to the vessels that move the blood flow into the aneurysm. Thus, temporary clipping is usually referred to the apposition of the temporary clip on the afferent vessels in order to stop the anterograde blood flow. However, since the blood could flow into the aneurysm retrogradely through the efferent vessels, it could be needed the application of temporary clip on these vessels in case of persisting bleeding [12, 15]. Therefore, proximal control is referred to the exposition of the afferent vessels, distal control of the efferent vessels [12]. The application of temporary clip is useful in case of complex aneurysm, to facilitate the dissection without risk of bleeding. Moreover, arresting the flow, temporary clipping led the aneurysm to soften, allowing an easier dissection for the visualization of the parent vessels [16].

Temporary clipping is also a savage maneuver in case of aneurysm rupture because it stops the blood flow into the aneurysm, facilitating the dissection of the parent vessels and the neck, allowing the application of the permanent clip [15, 17].

DOI: http://dx.doi.org/10.5772/intechopen.110774

Aneurysms with a single afferent vessel, or with multiple afferent and efferent vessels, could be classified. For this reason, different vessels should be exposed during the surgery considering aneurysm location:

- Middle cerebral artery (MCA) aneurysm:
    - Proximal control: sphenoidal segment of MCA (tract M1)
    - Distal control: post-bifurcation segments (tract M2–M3)
- Anterior communicating artery (ACoA) aneurysm:
    - Proximal control: precommunicating segment of anterior cerebral artery (tract A1) of both sides
    - Distal control: postcommunicating segments of anterior cerebral artery (tract A2) of both sides
- Pericallosal artery (PCaA) aneurysm:
    - Proximal control: precallosal (tract A3) or supracallosal (tract A4) segments of anterior cerebral artery, in relation to aneurysm location
    - Distal control: supracallosal (tract A4) or postcallosal (tract A5) segments of anterior cerebral artery, in relation to aneurysm location
- Posterior communicating artery (PCoA) aneurysm:
    - Proximal control: ophthalmic segments (tract C6) of internal carotid artery (ICA). Ophthalmic segments begins from the distal dural ring and end at the origin of PCoA.
    - Distal control: communicating segments (tract C7) of ICA, PCoA. Communicating segments begins from the origin of PCoA and ends at ICA bifurcation.
- Ophthalmic artery (OphA) aneurysm:
    - Proximal control: clinoidal segments (tract C5, which is the tract between the proximal and the distal dural ring) and ophthalmic segments (tract C6) of ICA, exposed through anterior clinoidectomy.
    - Distal control: supraclinoidal segments (tract C6-ophtalmic and C7-communicating) of ICA, OphA and PCoA.
- Basilar artery (BA) aneurysm:
    - Proximal control: basilar artery (BA)
    - Distal control: precommunicating segment (tract P1) of posterior cerebral artery (PCA), superior cerebellar artery (SCA)
- Posterior Inferior Cerebellar Artery (PICA) aneurysm:
    - Proximal control: vertebral artery (VA), anterior medullary segment (trac p1), lateral medullary segments (tract p2), tonsillomedullary segment (tract p3), or telovelotonsillar segments (tract p4) of PICA, in relation to aneurysm location

- ○ Distal control: anterior medullary segment (trac p1), lateral medullary segments (tract p2), tonsillomedullary segment (tract p3), or telovelotonsillar segments (tract p4) of PICA, in relation to aneurysm location

2.2 Permanent clipping

The application of a permanent clip requires the perfect knowledge of aneurysm anatomy, which should follow the Rothon rules [18]:

- Rule 1: aneurysms develop at sites where the parent artery branches off, which may be the origin of a side branch or a bifurcation

- Rule 2: aneurysm develops at hemodynamically stressful turns or curves in the artery's outer wall

- Rule 3: aneurysm points in the direction that blood would have flowed if the aneurysm site's curve had not been presented

- Rule 4: aneurysm is connected to a set of perforating arteries that (must be preserved)

Different clipping techniques have been described: simple clipping and multiple clipping.

Simple clipping refers to using a single clip for aneurysms with narrow neck and uncomplicated anatomy. It requires the use of the optimal clip in relation to neck conformation and size, considering that the application of the clip pressing the neck will increase its length and that the final part of the blade should cross the neck [12].

Multiple clipping is a technique that allows the application of more than one clip to close the neck of the aneurysm in sequential steps, and it is usually adopted to treat aneurysms with complex anatomy, including intersecting clips, stacked clips, and overlapping clips [12]. *Intersecting clipping* technique describes the application of the second clip angled into the first clip and intersecting it, thus allowing the remodeling of the aneurysm with a *bleb* that otherwise would be impossible to exclude with a simple clipping (**Figure 1A**) [19, 20].

Stacked clipping consists of the application of clips in the same direction and parallel to each other, in which usually the first one closes the aneurism, and the other ones closes the remnant *of the neck* beneath to the first clip (understacked). In case of application of the first clip on the neck, if another clip is necessary over the first one to complete the closure, this is defined overstacked (**Figure 1B**) [12, 20, 21].

Overlapping clipping describes the application of a second fenestrated clip over a first straight clip encircling it, in order to close a distal remnant beneath the initial clip (**Figure 1C**) [12, 20].

Tandem clipping is the technique described by Drake, which consists of the application of a first straight fenestrated clip to close the distal aneurysm (encircling in the fenestration a parent vessel), and a second clip to close the fenestration (**Figure 1D**) [12, 20, 21].

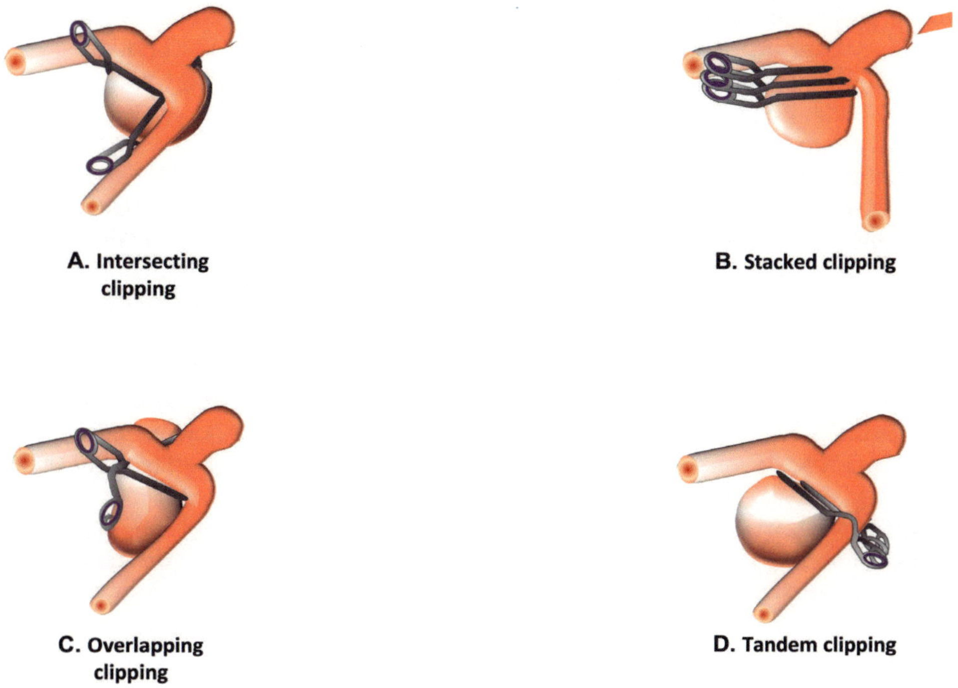

Figure 1.
The figure depicts the most common techniques for permanent clipping of cerebral aneurysms.

3. Intraoperative strategies to detect aneurysm obliteration and parent vessels patency

3.1 Micro-Doppler ultrasonography (MUSG)

Doppler ultrasonography was first employed to assess cerebral hemodynamics in extracranial arteries. This method was further refined for the transcranial examination of brain vessels [22]. Technological advancements allowed the reduction of the ultrasound probe's size by raising the ultrasonic frequency. Microprobes for the direct examination of small brain vessels were created as a result of further research [23–25].

Before and after the aneurysm clipping, blood flow velocities in the aneurysm sac and the nearby arteries could be measured using intraoperative microvascular Doppler ultrasonography (MUSG). The probe with a 1 mm-diameter pulsed wave mode is used to make the Doppler measurements. In addition, a suction cannula could be used to insert the Doppler probe, thus allowing precise positioning and stability. With an insonation angle of 30 to 60 degrees, the probe is used to examine all exposed arteries close to the aneurysm as well as the aneurysmal sac [26].

MUSG was first described by Lanborde et al. for intraoperative monitoring of large cerebral aneurysms [27]. MUSG has the ability to identify the orientation and hemodynamics of the parent arteries, as well as the vortex flow or thrombus within the aneurysm sac, prior to the positioning of clip. Particularly in large and challenging aneurysm surgery, MUSG monitoring could determine if the aneurysm sac is entirely clipped and whether parent or perforating arteries are stenosed or accidentally clipped. MUSG can detect all vessels in the Wills circle and its branches, including those with a diameter of less than 1 mm, because of the availability of a high-frequency micro-probe [28].

Bailes et al. [28] investigated the use of MUSG in aneurysm surgery, observing a capability to detect occlusion or stenosis of parent vessels in 31% of cases after clip positioning, and therefore allowing immediate adjusting.

Stendel et al. [26] MUSG discovered a meaningful stenosis of an adjacent artery caused by clip location in 17 out of 90 (18.9%) aneurysms. In addition, 11 out of 90 (12.2%) patients evaluated with Doppler ultrasound showed a predominantly unoccluded aneurysm. In 26 out of 90 (28.8%) patients, the aneurysm clip was repositioned based on the MDUG findings.

In conclusion, the complete closure of cerebral aneurysms and the patency of parent arteries, arterial branches, and main perforators could be documented by intraoperative MUSG, which is safe, rapid, efficient, dependable, and economical tool. In many situations, this method can be utilized safely in addition to other tools to monitor surgical aneurysms, reducing the risk of postoperative cerebral stroke. The limitations of MUSG include its vulnerability to changes in detecting angle and depth, fluid surrounding vessels, and tractor, as well as its inability to detect the aneurysm's back or minute remnant of its neck.

3.2 Indocyanine green video angiography (ICG-VA)

In 1956, the United States Food and Drug Administration (FDA) approved the use of indocyanine green (ICG) dye, a near-infrared (NIR) fluorescent tricarbocya-9 dye, to assess liver and cardiocirculatory functions. Ophthalmic angiography received additional FDA approval in 1975. ICG dye has an absorption and emission peak (805 and 835 nm, respectively) within the "optical window" of tissue, where endogenous chromophores have minimal absorption. After intravenous administration, ICG primarily binds to globulins (1 lipo-proteins) within 1 to 2 seconds. There is typical vascular permeability, and the dye is still intravascular. The liver is the only organ in the body that can excrete the indocyanine green dye, which has a plasma half-life of 3 to 4 minutes. ICG dye should be administered for video angiography (VA) at a dose of 0.2 to 0.5 mg/kg, with a daily maximum dose of 5 mg/kg.

The use of intraoperative NIR VA was first described by Raabe et al. in 2003, where ICG dye was used for intraoperative observation of vascular flow [29]. A light source that has a wavelength covering a portion of the ICG absorption band illuminates the operating field from the microscope (range 700–850 nm, maximum 805 nm). A bolus of the ICG dye is administered via peripheral vein (the standard 25-mg dose dissolved in 5 ml of water), and a nonintensified video camera captures the fluorescence (spectral range 780–950 nm, maximum 835 nm). To exclusively collect ICG-induced fluorescence, ambient and excitation light are blocked using an optical filter. As a result, real-time viewing of venous, capillary, and artery angiographic pictures is possible [30].

Some authors compared intraoperative and postoperative findings on the patency of the parent, branching, and perforating arteries and the clip occlusion of the aneurysm as indicated by ICG-VA, with the standard digital subtractive (DS) angiography. They observed that in 90% of cases, the results of ICG-VA matched those of intra and postoperative DS angiography. In 7.3% of patients, the ICG method failed to detect a modest but hemodynamically insignificant stenosis that was visible on

DS angiography. In three cases, the ICG approach failed to pick up angiographically significant findings. In two of the cases, the missed findings had no clinical or surgical repercussions; in the third, a 4-mm residual neck may necessitate additional surgery. In 9% of cases, indocyanine green VA gave the surgeon useful information about clip repair [30].

In 90% of instances, the results of ICG-VA matched those of intra- and post-operative DS angiography. In 7.3% of patients, the ICG method failed to detect a modest but hemodynamically insignificant stenosis that was visible on DS angiography. In three cases (one hemodynamically important stenosis and two residual aneurysm necks [2.7% of cases]), the ICG approach failed to pick up angiographically significant findings. In two of the cases, the missed findings had no clinical or surgical repercussions; in the third, a 4-mm residual neck may necessitate additional surgery. A substantial amount of information was provided to the surgeon using indocyanine green VA. The authors concluded that ICG-VA using a microscope is easy to perform and gives real-time data on the aneurysm sac and the patency of all diameters of arteries.

Many others studied compared the safety and efficacy of ICG-VA with DS angiography [1, 5, 13, 14, 17, 19, 20, 31, 32].

Ozgiray et al. [5] described that in 93.5% of aneurysms ICG-VA accurately determined vascular patency and aneurysm obliteration; only in 3.6% of cases ICG-VA showed no flow after clipping whereas puncturing the aneurysm's dome indicated residual flow, in 0.9% it demonstrated sustained flow within the aneurysm in one whereas MUSG and puncture of the dome did not, and in 0.9% it failed to show residual neck.

Della Puppa et al. [13] analyzed the role of ICG-VA added to the other techniques, observing that ICG-VA was useful for detecting parent vessels occlusion or residual aneurysm in 8.3% of cases. Moreover, only one false negative remnant neck was noted, with a negative predictive value of 98.8%, and ICG-VA was more sensitive to reveal remnant primarily in atherosclerotic aneurysms ($P < 0.05$).

In conclusion, ICG VA represents the best tool to directly observe parent vessels patency and aneurysm obliteration. The surgical microscope's integration and its ability to show perforating arteries with submillimeter widths are two of its distinctive advantages. Its utility during aneurysm surgery is supported by its ease use, rapidity, and high level of accuracy for identifying partially clipped aneurysms and accidentally occluded vessels. Moreover, the ICG-VA has the potential to be more broadly accessible than intraoperative DS angiography.

3.3 Electrophysiological monitoring

Electroencephalography (EEG), motor evoked potentials (MEPs), somatosensory evoked potentials (SSEPs), visual evoked potentials (VEPs), and auditory evoked potentials are few of the intraoperative neuromonitoring (IONM) techniques available for cerebrovascular surgery. The overall objective of each modality is to improve the patient's functional outcome by detecting changes in brain activity that can indicate possible neurological compromise. Each modality has its own unique applications [33, 34]. Electrophysiological monitoring is useful to observe potential early ischemia during temporary clipping or after permanent clipping, allowing to remove of the temporary clip to restore the flow, or to explore the parent and perforating vessels after permanent clip detecting a possible erroneous clipping [15, 35].

Usually, the motor pathway is monitored by stimulating the motor area using electrodes inserted in C1–C2 (C3–C4) through a train of 4 to 5 stimuli with the intensity of 250 to 500 Hz. The somatosensory pathway is monitored by stimulating contralateral medianus nerve at the wrist for the upper limb SSEPs, and the contralateral tibial nerve at the medial malleolus for the lower limb SSEPs. General anesthesia could affect the results of IONM; thus, total intravenous anesthesia is recommended, possibly avoiding the use of neuromuscular blockers unless absolutely necessary [13, 36].

Knowing the N20 peak's amplitude in relation to the evoked parietal response is crucial. N20 peak amplitude was decreased by more than 50% when compared to its absolute values, indicating a decrease in rCBF values of around 12–16 mL/100 g/min. This is comparable to cerebral ischemia that may be reversible, however, chronic maintenance of a low rCBF may result in cerebral infarct [37, 38].

Penchet et al. observed a significant reduction of SSEP (more than 50%) in 25.9% of the patients, of which 6.9% with postoperative ischemic stroke and partial or no recovery, 19% with complete recovery, and only two postoperative ischemic strokes. The authors concluded that changes in SSEP had a strong correlation with postoperative stroke incidence [34].

Staarmann et al. [36] described IONM alterations in 15 cases out of 133 clipped aneurysms, including 12 transient changes without new postoperative deficits and 3 permanent changes with new postoperative deficits. Transcranial motor evoked potentials and somatosensory evoked potentials predicted 2 and 1 of the postoperative deficits, respectively. Moreover, they observed only 1.1% incidence of IONM alterations and permanent neurological deficits associated with temporary clipping [36].

Della Puppa et al. [13] observed a reduction of evoked potential in 11 patients during temporary or permanent clipping, 10 in accordance with MEPs, and 1 in accordance with SSEP. All these IONM normalized after temporary clip removal or permanent clip repositioning. MEP was significantly correlated with proximal located aneurysm (ACoA, ICA, M1).

In conclusion, multimodal IONM is very sensitive and specific for identifying new deficits. The early detection of potential reversible ischemia allows maneuvers such as temporary clipping removal or the identification of another component (such as releasing brain retraction or reposition of permanent clip) to lower the likelihood of postoperative complications.

4. Future perspectives

ICG-VA represents the most dominant innovation of the latest years for the surgical treatment of brain aneurysms. Future technological advances should potentially allow to facilitate three-dimensional (3D) orientation, optimize clip placement, and manage the proximal and distal control [39].

One of the first considerations that it could be done about future advances in vascular neurosurgery is that brain aneurysm surgery represents a specific technical challenge for young neurosurgeons, due to the huge increase in endovascular technology in the latest years. Since endovascular treatments continue to develop, a similar focus on technological innovation in open surgical repair should be implemented, for patients to continue to benefit from whichever treatment option is most effective for their aneurysm. Thus, training in this subspeciality of neurosurgery represents an increasing challenge in the modern era and a specific field that applies to increased learning opportunities [40]. High-fidelity surgical simulators may provide a partial answer by enabling surgeons to gain expertise. In fact, preoperative simulation tailored to the patient who will be operated, as well as 3D models, could be detrimental to compensate for the lack of opportunities to learn vascular surgery, leading young neurosurgeons to an easier improvement of technical skills, thus facilitating 3D orientation and optimizing the management of surgical procedures [41].

Another issue to be considered regarding future advances is the identification of technologies that would improve clip application (e.g., advances in applicators, advances in clips) and intraoperative visualization (e.g., endoscopes and intraoperative imaging). Endoscopes are not usually included in the aneurysm surgical workflow, but they could improve the visualization of aneurysm "blind spot", facilitating aneurysm management and 3D orientation [39].

Hybrid operating theaters, which include intraoperative CT scans and intraoperative angiography, are not very diffused. Still, they should be identified as potential future advances to optimize clip application and 3D orientation, increasing the safety of aneurysm obliteration and neck reconstruction, reducing surgical morbidity despite of the reduced surgical cases compared to the past.

In conclusion, the majority of future advances in vascular neurosurgery should be targeted to optimize clip application and improve 3D visualization and orientation, for example, increasing the use of endoscopic-assisted surgery, implementing the development of surgical simulators, and investing in the growth of hybrid opened-endovascular technique thanks to hybrid operating theaters [39].

5. Conclusions

Microsurgical obliteration of cerebral aneurysms represents the best long-term treatment for this pathology. Despite high surgical expertise, aneurysm surgery is often associated with an increased risk of intraoperative rupture. For this reason, vascular control is pivotal and should be aimed at by the neurosurgeon during aneurysm surgery. The application of single or multiple definitive clips on the neck of the aneurysm can be achieved with different techniques in order to arrest the blood flow into the dome [12]. Intraoperative use of ICG-VA, MUSG, and IONM can effectively reduce brain tissue ischemia ad morbidity after clipping intracranial aneurysm, thus improving the surgical outcome. Microsurgical clipping with the use of a multimodal monitoring method led to a high incidence of aneurysm exclusion with little morbidity [13].

Conflict of interest

The authors declare no conflict of inte 3rest.

Acronyms and abbreviations

SAH	subarachnoid hemorrhage
MUSG	Micro-Doppler ultrasonography
ICG-VA	indocyanine green video angiography
IONM	electrophysiological neuromonitoring
MCA	Middle cerebral artery aneurysm

ACoA	Anterior communicating artery
PCaA	Pericallosal artery
PCoA	Posterior communicating artery
OphA	Ophthalmic artery
BA	basilar artery
PICA	Posterior Inferior Cerebellar Artery
ICA	internal carotid artery
FDA	Food and Drug Administration
ICG	indocyanine green
NIR	near-infrared
VA	video angiography
DS	digital subtractive
EEG	Electroencephalography
MEPs	motor evoked potentials
SSEPs	somatosensory evoked potentials
VEPs	visual evoked potentials
CBF	cerebral blood flow
3D	three-dimensional

Author details

Pasquale Anania[1*] and Pietro Fiaschi[1,2]

1 Department of Neurosurgery, IRCCS Ospedale Policlinico San Martino, Genoa, Italy

2 Department of Neurosciences, Rehabilitation, Ophthalmology, Genetics, Maternal and Child Health, University of Genoa, Genoa, Italy

*Address all correspondence to: pasquale.anania@hsanmartino.it

References

[1] Li Z, Zhang G, Huang G, Wang Z, Tan H, Liu J, et al. Intraoperative combined use of somatosensory evoked potential, microvascular Doppler sonography, and Indocyanine green angiography in clipping of intracranial aneurysm. Medical Science Monitor. 2016;**22**:373-379. DOI: 10.12659/MSM.895457

[2] Zhong Z, Sun Y, Lin D, Sun Q, Bian L. Surgical treatment of brain tumor coexisted with intracranial aneurysm—Case series and review of the literature. Neurosurgical Review. 2013;**36**:645-656. DOI: 10.1007/s10143-013-0477-7

[3] Molyneux A, Kerr R. International Subarachnoid Aneurysm Trial (ISAT) of neurosurgical clipping versus endovascular coiling in 2143 patients with ruptured intracranial aneurysms: A randomized trial. Journal of Stroke and Cerebrovascular Diseases. 2002;**11**:304-314. DOI: 10.1053/jscd.2002.130390

[4] Farag E, Ebrahim Z, Traul D, Katzan I, Manno E. Perioperative management of intracranial aneurysm and subarachnoid hemorrhage. Current Pharmaceutical Design. 2013;**19**:5792-5808. DOI: 10.2174/1381612811319990062

[5] Özgiray E, Aktüre E, Patel N, Baggott C, Bozkurt M, Niemann D, et al. How reliable and accurate is indocyanine green video angiography in the evaluation of aneurysm obliteration? Clinical Neurology and Neurosurgery. 2013;**115**:870-878. DOI: 10.1016/j.clineuro.2012.08.027

[6] Mery FJ, Amin-Hanjani S, Charbel FT. Is an angiographically obliterated aneurysm always secure? Neurosurgery. 2008;**62**:979-982. DOI: 10.1227/01.neu.0000318190.63901.62

[7] de Oliveira JG, Beck J, Seifert V, Teixeira MJ, Raabe A. Assessment of flow in perforating arteries during intracranial aneurysm surgery using intraoperative near-infrared indocyanine green videoangiography. Operative Neurosurgery. 2007;**61**:63-73. DOI: 10.1227/01.neu.0000289715.18297.08

[8] Dashti R, Laakso A, Niemelä M, Porras M, Hernesniemi J. Microscope-integrated near-infrared indocyanine green videoangiography during surgery of intracranial aneurysms: The Helsinki experience. Surgical Neurology. 2009;**71**:543-550. DOI: 10.1016/j.surneu.2009.01.027

[9] Dashti R, Laakso A, Niemelä M, Porras M, Celik Ö, Navratil O, et al. Application of microscope integrated indocyanine green video-angiography during microneurosurgical treatment of intracranial aneurysms: A review. Acta Neurochirurgica Supplement. 2010:107-109. DOI: 10.1007/978-3-211-99373-6_17

[10] Fischer G, Stadie A, Oertel JMK. Near-infrared indocyanine green videoangiography versus microvascular Doppler sonography in aneurysm surgery. Acta Neurochirurgica. 2010;**152**:1519-1525. DOI: 10.1007/s00701-010-0723-5

[11] Shim J-H, Yoon S-M, Bae H-G, Yun I-G, Shim J-J, Lee K-S, et al. Which treatment modality is more injurious to the brain in patients with subarachnoid Hemorrhage? Degree of brain damage assessed by serum S100 protein after aneurysm clipping or coiling. Cerebrovascular Diseases. 2012;**34**:38-47. DOI: 10.1159/000338786

[12] Lawton MT. Seven Aneurysms: Tenets and Techniques for Clipping. New York: Thieme Medical Publishers; 2011

[13] della Puppa A, Rossetto M, Volpin F, Rustemi O, Grego A, Gerardi A, et al. Microsurgical clipping of intracranial aneurysms assisted by neurophysiological monitoring, microvascular flow probe, and ICG-VA: Outcomes and intraoperative data on a multimodal strategy. World Neurosurgery. 2018;**113**:e336-e344. DOI: 10.1016/j.wneu.2018.02.029

[14] Hammer A, Steiner A, Kerry G, Ranaie G, Baer I, Hammer CM, et al. Treatment of ruptured intracranial aneurysms yesterday and now. PLoS One. 2017;**12**:e0172837. DOI: 10.1371/journal.pone.0172837

[15] Charbel FT, Ausman JI, Diaz FG, Malik GM, Dujovny M, Sanders J. Temporary clipping in aneurysm surgery: Technique and results. Surgical Neurology. 1991;**36**:83-90. DOI: 10.1016/0090-3019(91)90223-V

[16] Malinova V, Schatlo B, Voit M, Suntheim P, Rohde V, Mielke D. The impact of temporary clipping during aneurysm surgery on the incidence of delayed cerebral ischemia after aneurysmal subarachnoid hemorrhage. Journal of Neurosurgery. 2018;**129**:84-90. DOI: 10.3171/2017.3.JNS162505

[17] Lawton MT, Du R. Effect of the Neurosurgeon's surgical experience on outcomes from intraoperative aneurysmal rupture. Neurosurgery. 2005;**57**:9-15. DOI: 10.1227/01.NEU.0000163082.20941.EF

[18] Rothon AL. Rhoton's Cranial Anatomy and Surgical Approaches. 1st ed. Philadelphia, US: Lippincott Williams & Wilkins; 2007

[19] Sanai N, Caldwell N, Englot DJ, Lawton MT. Advanced technical skills are required for microsurgical clipping of posterior communicating artery aneurysms in the endovascular era. Neurosurgery. 2012;**71**:285-295. DOI: 10.1227/NEU.0b013e318256c3eb

[20] Kamide T, Burkhardt J-K, Tabani H, Safaee M, Lawton MT. Microsurgical clipping techniques and outcomes for Paraclinoid internal carotid artery aneurysms. Operative Neurosurgery. 2020;**18**:183-192. DOI: 10.1093/ons/opz157

[21] del Maestro RF. Origin of the drake fenestrated aneurysm clip. Journal of Neurosurgery. 2000;**92**:1056-1064. DOI: 10.3171/jns.2000.92.6.1056

[22] Aaslid R, Markwalder T-M, Nornes H. Noninvasive transcranial Doppler ultrasound recording of flow velocity in basal cerebral arteries. Journal of Neurosurgery. 1982;**57**:769-774. DOI: 10.3171/jns.1982.57.6.0769

[23] Gilsbach JM, Hassler WE. Intraoperative doppler and real time sonography in neurosurgery. Neurosurgical Review. 1984;**7**:199-208. DOI: 10.1007/BF01780705

[24] Gilsbach J. Mikrovaskuläre intraoperative Doppler-Sonographie. Ultraschall in der Medizin. 2008;**5**:246-254. DOI: 10.1055/s-2007-1012102

[25] Nornes H, Grip A, Wikeby P. Intraoperative evaluation of cerebral hemodynamics using directional Doppler technique. Journal of Neurosurgery. 1979;**50**:570-577. DOI: 10.3171/jns.1979.50.5.0570

[26] Stendel R. Intraoperative microvascular Doppler ultrasonography in cerebral aneurysm surgery. Journal of Neurology, Neurosurgery, and Psychiatry. 2000;**68**:29-35. DOI: 10.1136/jnnp.68.1.29

[27] Laborde G, Gilsbach J, Harders A. The Microvascular Doppler — an

Intraoperative Tool for the Treatment of Large and Giant Aneurysms. In: Proceedings of the 8th European Congress of Neurosurgery Barcelona, September 6-11, 1987. Vienna: Springer Vienna; 1988. pp. 75-80. DOI: 10.1007/978-3-7091-8975-7_15

[28] Bailes JE, Tantuwaya LS, Fukushima T, Schurman GW, Davis D. Intraoperative microvascular Doppler sonography in aneurysm surgery. Neurosurgery. 1997;**40**:965-972. DOI: 10.1097/00006123-199705000-00018

[29] Raabe A, Beck J, Gerlach R, Zimmermann M, Seifert V. Near-infrared Indocyanine green video angiography: A new method for intraoperative assessment of vascular flow. Neurosurgery. 2003;**52**:132-139. DOI: 10.1097/00006123-200301000-00017

[30] Raabe A, Nakaji P, Beck J, Kim LJ, Hsu FPK, Kamerman JD, et al. Prospective evaluation of surgical microscope—Integrated intraoperative near-infrared indocyanine green videoangiography during aneurysm surgery. Journal of Neurosurgery. 2005;**103**:982-989. DOI: 10.3171/jns.2005.103.6.0982

[31] Norat P, Soldozy S, Elsarrag M, Sokolowski J, Yağmurlu K, Park MS, et al. Application of Indocyanine green Videoangiography in aneurysm surgery: Evidence, techniques, practical tips. Frontiers in Surgery. 2019;**2019**:6. DOI: 10.3389/fsurg.2019.00034

[32] Roessler K, Krawagna M, Dörfler A, Buchfelder M, Ganslandt O. Essentials in intraoperative indocyanine green videoangiography assessment for intracranial aneurysm surgery: Conclusions from 295 consecutively clipped aneurysms and review of the literature. Neurosurgical Focus. 2014;**36**:E7. DOI: 10.3171/2013.11.FOCUS13475

[33] Szelényi A, Langer D, Kothbauer K, de Camargo AB, Flamm ES, Deletis V. Monitoring of muscle motor evoked potentials during cerebral aneurysm surgery: Intraoperative changes and postoperative outcome. Journal of Neurosurgery. 2006;**105**:675-681. DOI: 10.3171/jns.2006.105.5.675

[34] Penchet G, Arné P, Cuny E, Monteil P, Loiseau H, Castel J-P. Use of intraoperative monitoring of somatosensory evoked potentials to prevent ischaemic stroke after surgical exclusion of middle cerebral artery aneurysms. Acta Neurochirurgica. 2007;**149**:357-364. DOI: 10.1007/s00701-007-1119-z

[35] Samson D, Batjer HH, Bowman G, Mootz L, Krippner WJ, Meyer YJ, et al. A clinical study of the parameters and effects of temporary arterial occlusion in the management of intracranial aneurysms. Neurosurgery. 1994;**34**:22-28; discussion 28-9

[36] Staarmann B, O'Neal K, Magner M, Zuccarello M. Sensitivity and specificity of intraoperative Neuromonitoring for identifying safety and duration of temporary aneurysm clipping based on vascular territory, a multimodal strategy. World Neurosurgery. 2017;**100**:522-530. DOI: 10.1016/j.wneu.2017.01.009

[37] Symon L. The relationship between CBF, evoked potentials and the clinical features in cerebral ischaemia. Acta Neurologica Scandinavica. Supplementum. 1980;**78**:175-190

[38] Lesnick JE, Michele JJ, Simeone FA, DeFeo S, Welsh FA. Alteration of somatosensory evoked potentials in response to global ischemia. Journal of

Neurosurgery. 1984;**60**:490-494. DOI: 10.3171/jns.1984.60.3.0490

[39] Muirhead WR, Layard Horsfall H, Khan DZ, Koh C, Grover PJ, Toma AK, et al. Microsurgery for intracranial aneurysms: A qualitative survey on technical challenges and technological solutions. Frontiers in Surgery. 2022;**2022**:9. DOI: 10.3389/fsurg.2022.957450

[40] Burkhardt J-K, Lawton MT. Training young neurosurgeons in open microsurgical aneurysm treatment. World Neurosurgery. 2017;**103**:919-920. DOI: 10.1016/j.wneu.2017.04.089

[41] Liu Y, Gao Q, Du S, Chen Z, Fu J, Chen B, et al. Fabrication of cerebral aneurysm simulator with a desktop 3D printer. Scientific Reports. 2017;**7**:44301. DOI: 10.1038/srep44301

Chapter 7

Perspective Chapter: Role of Direct Surgery for Recurrent Aneurysms after Endovascular Treatment

Tsuyoshi Izumo

Abstract

Treatment strategies for cerebral aneurysms have changed dramatically in recent years with advances in endovascular therapy. Advances in devices, endovascular surgeons' skills, and diagnostic modalities have improved the results of endovascular treatment, making it a safer and more reliable treatment option. On the other hand, we are encountering an increasing number of cases of postoperative recurrence. Direct surgery has a specific role in treating these recurrent cases, and it has become essential to establish a decision-making method and surgical technique for treating these cases. In this chapter, I will discuss the treatment options for recurrent cerebral aneurysms after endovascular treatment and the practical application of direct clipping and bypass surgery.

Keywords: cerebral aneurysms, direct surgery, endovascular treatment, recurrence, neurosurgery

1. Introduction

Direct surgery for recurrent cerebral aneurysms after endovascular treatment is complicated, and great care must be taken in determining its indications. In addition, the actual procedure often requires technical ingenuity. In this chapter, we will discuss in detail the role of direct surgery for this aneurysm and its surgical innovations.

2. History of treatment for intracranial aneurysms

The history of craniotomy clipping for cerebral aneurysms is long. Dandy WE reported clipping surgery using a V-shaped malleable clip in 1937 [1]. Many papers have been published since 1959 when Mount LA et al. reported a procedure using the highly operable Selverstone clamp [2]. Since then, craniotomy clipping results have improved with the advent of the latest cerebral aneurysm clips and surgeon skill improvements. Many neurosurgeons have accepted this as a highly reliable long-term procedure with a low recurrence rate for unruptured and ruptured cerebral aneurysms [3–5]. The most significant advantage of this treatment is that it immediately removes the cerebral aneurysm from the general circulatory system, leading to a very low probability of rupture or rerupture. On the other hand, it is necessarily a relatively invasive procedure because it involves skin and muscle incisions, craniotomy, and subdural brain manipulation, making it a burdensome procedure for patients with medical complications and the elderly. Minimally invasive surgical techniques centered on key hole surgery have been developed to solve this problem, and patient satisfaction has improved, and it has also been reported to reduce the frequency of cerebral vasospasm in subarachnoid hemorrhage cases and to improve treatment prognosis [6–9].

Endovascular treatment as a counterpart to cranial clipping as a treatment for cerebral aneurysms was reported as early as 1832. It was intended to occlude the aneurysm by wire insertion or electrothrombosis. Still, it was not used to occlude intracranial arteries. The most significant disadvantages of endovascular treatment are its high rate of complications such as distal embolism, high mortality rate, and the long time required for occlusion [10]. Subsequently, treatment of large and giant cavernous sinus internal carotid artery aneurysms using a detachable balloon was reported by Serbienko and colleagues. Since then, many good treatment results have been reported with improvements and performance enhancements by Romadanov, Debrun, Hieshima, and Taki [11–14]. Conversely, they are challenging to apply to intradural cerebral aneurysms and new devices have been awaited.

Endovascular treatment of cerebral aneurysms has made great strides since the introduction of the Guglielmi Detachable Coil (GDC) in 1991 [15]. Compared to conventional devices, this is an electrically detachable platinum coil, easy to operate, and incredibly soft, making it less invasive to the aneurysm wall, enabling safer and more reliable endovascular treatment of intracranial aneurysms. The GDC received FDA approval in 1995. Since then, the GDC has become a widely used treatment for cerebral aneurysms. The International Subarachnoid Aneurysm Trial (ISAT), a randomized controlled trial of coil embolization versus surgical clipping for ruptured cerebral arterial aneurysms, was published in 2002 [16]. The results showed that in patients in whom endovascular coiling and neurosurgical clipping were the treatment of choice for ruptured intracranial aneurysms, the 1-year disability-free survival rate was significantly better with endovascular coiling. The long-term risk of rebleeding from treated aneurysms was also lower for both treatment modalities but was suggested to be slightly more frequent with endovascular coiling [16]. Since the publication of this report, coil embolization has become a more aggressive option for ruptured and unruptured cerebral aneurysms, especially in Europe and the United States. Furthermore, the Barrow Ruptured Aneurysm Trial (BRAT), which compared coil embolization and surgical clipping to treat ruptured cerebral aneurysms, confirmed that the treatment prognoses for both procedures were comparable [17, 18]. In a report from Australia covering cases from 2008 to 2018 based on the Australian National Hospital Morbidity database, endovascular treatment for cerebral aneurysms accounted for 58.4% of all cases [19]. Furthermore, the Nationwide Inpatient Sample database from 2002 to 2012 reported that in a total of 23,053 patients with unruptured cerebral aneurysms, coil embolization was the procedure of choice in approximately 73% of cases [20]. Opportunities for endovascular treatment options for cerebral aneurysms, coupled with advances in the technology of the devices and surgeons, will continue to increase in proportion.

3. The aneurysmal recurrence rate after endovascular coil embolization has improved but is still high

While endovascular treatment is a minimally invasive treatment for cerebral aneurysms, the biggest problem is that, unlike craniotomy clipping, which is a treatment that can completely exclude cerebral aneurysms from the circulatory system, it is a method of filling coils with aneurysms while they are still in the circulatory system, which inevitably results in a relatively high postoperative recurrence rate. According to the ISAT results, the cerebral aneurysm recurrence rate after endovascular treatment is reported to be 17.4% [16]. The BRAT results also reported a 15.6% cerebral aneurysm recurrence rate after 1 year of endovascular treatment [21]. According to reports on so-called real-world data from other than these randomized controlled trials, the recurrence rate is 20–30% [22, 23]. But recent reports indicate that the rate of cerebral aneurysm recurrence after endovascular treatment is trending downward, from 10% to the 5% range [24, 25]. This is primarily due to new technological innovations such as stent-assisted coil embolization. On the other hand, as mentioned above, the number of cerebral aneurysms treated endovascularly is increasing. As the population grows, it is clear that the number of aneurysms requiring retreatment will inevitably increase, no matter how low the recurrence rate becomes.

4. The rupture rate of recurrent aneurysms after endovascular coil embolization is low. What are the characteristics of the recurrence with a high risk of rupture?

The rupture rate of recurrent aneurysms after endovascular coil embolization is low. A systematic review by Arnaout OM et al. reported the risk of recurrent cerebral aneurysms after initial coil embolization of 2.3 to 8.3% or 0.8% per year [22]. A study by the CARAT Investigators of 1010 patients (299 after coil embolization) reported that the rate of delayed rebleeding from the recurrent aneurysm after coil embolization was 0.11% per year [26]. As these indicate, the risk of rupture of recurrent cerebral aneurysms after initial coil embolization is low. Thus, these are relatively stable lesions, and not all are indications of retreatment.

On the other hand, we have experienced cases of death or serious illness due to the rupture of these recurrent cerebral aneurysms, and we would like to call for caution.

We present a case of our own experience (**Figure 1**). The patient was a 63-year-old woman with a subarachnoid hemorrhage due to a ruptured basilar bifurcation aneurysm and underwent coil embolization at another hospital 3 years earlier. She was discharged home with a modified Rankin Scale score (mRS) of 0. During outpatient follow-up, a recurrence of the aneurysm, which had been treated for 3 years, was found, and the patient was referred to our outpatient clinic. Her neurological imaging study showed marked re-enlargement of the aneurysm due to coil compaction (**Figure 1a** and **b**), and we were considering coil embolization for retreatment of the aneurysm. However, 1 week after the visit, she suddenly developed a loss of consciousness and was brought into our emergency department. When she came to our hospital, she was in a coma with bilateral dilated pupils, and a head CT scan showed marked intraventricular hemorrhage and acute hydrocephalus (**Figure 1c**). She underwent emergency ventricular drainage, but the neurological findings did not improve even after the operation, and she died and was discharged from the hospital the day after arrival.

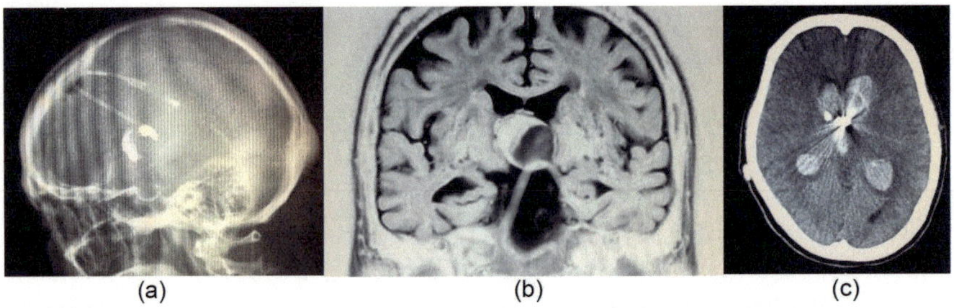

Figure 1.
(a)-(c), (a): Lateral view of a plain X-ray image of the head: The coil mass is divided into two pieces due to coil compaction. (b): Magnectin resonance imaging (MRI) coronal section of the head shows the recurrent partially thrombosed basilar bifurcation aneurysm. (c): A head computed tomography (CT) scan shows marked intraventricular hemorrhage and ventricular dilatation.

As this case demonstrates, clinicians must be fully aware of the possibility of recurrent cerebral aneurysms that can rupture and cause death or serious clinical consequences. So what are the characteristics of recurrent cerebral aneurysms are most likely to lead to rupture?

What are the characteristics of recurrent cerebral aneurysms after endovascular treatment with a high risk of bleeding?

1. It has been reported that progressive growing aneurysms are at high risk for hemorrhage [27].

2. The rebleeding rate of cerebral aneurysms with recurrent filling is reported to be 7.9% over 5 years [28].

3. Recurrent aneurysms with fundal migration of coil loops mean a dynamic inflammatory process is involved, and a high bleeding rate has been reported [29].

4. A high rebleeding rate of 17.6% has been reported when the occlusion rate after coil embolization is less than 70% [26]. In such recurrent cerebral aneurysms after coil embolization, as described above, the risk of severe subarachnoid hemorrhage due to bleeding is considered high. Thus, aggressive treatment should be recommended in these cases.

5. Role of direct surgery for recurrent aneurysms after endovascular coil embolization

The treatment selection for recurrent cerebral aneurysms after endovascular treatment should be based on an individualization policy. However, the difficulty of direct surgery is high in these aneurysms because of coil mass extrusion, thrombus formation in the aneurysms, adhesion to vital cranial nerves and branches due to inflammatory changes in the aneurysm wall, thickening of the aneurysm wall, and coil loop scarring to the parent artery. On the other hand, endovascular treatment is often relatively easy to retreat. Therefore, endovascular retreatment is the first choice to treat recurrent cerebral aneurysms after endovascular treatment safely.

Is endovascular treatment the optimal retreatment strategy for all patients with recurrent cerebral aneurysms after endovascular treatment? The recurrence rate of cerebral aneurysms after initial endovascular treatment has been reported to range from 4.7 to 17.4% [30–32]. On the other hand, the re-recurrence rate of endovascular retreated recurrent aneurysms has been reported to have a high cerebral aneurysm recurrence rate ranging from 44.1 to 48.8% [32–34]. Therefore, if endovascular retreatment is chosen for all post-endovascular recurrent cerebral aneurysms, the reoccurrence rate will inevitably be high, and multiple retreatments may sometimes be required. Although endovascular retreatment is a relatively safe and easy treatment for recurrent cerebral aneurysms after initial endovascular treatment, we should be careful not to choose this treatment method too easily.

It has been reported that the recurrence rate of endovascular treatment of recurrent cerebral aneurysms after initial endovascular treatment varies greatly depending on the mechanisms of recurrence (**Figure 2**). When endovascular treatment was selected for recurrent cerebral aneurysms after initial endovascular treatment, the multiple re-coiling rates for patients with recurrence by the coil compaction mechanism was 21.3%. The multiple re-coiling rates for patients with recurrence by the regrowth mechanism were extremely high at 85.7% [29]. Therefore, choosing direct surgery for recurrent cerebral aneurysms with a regrowth mechanism is crucial to minimize the multiple recurrences.

In addition, the flow diverter is now available as a new option for treating recurrent cerebral aneurysms after initial coil embolization. In a study comparing the pipeline embolization device (PED: 18 patients) and coil embolization for recurrent aneurysms after initial coil embolization, the complication rate was similar for PED and coil embolization, and the recurrence rate was significantly lower for PED than for coil embolization ($p < 0.037$) [35]. Moreover, in a study of flow diverter treatment (17 patients) for

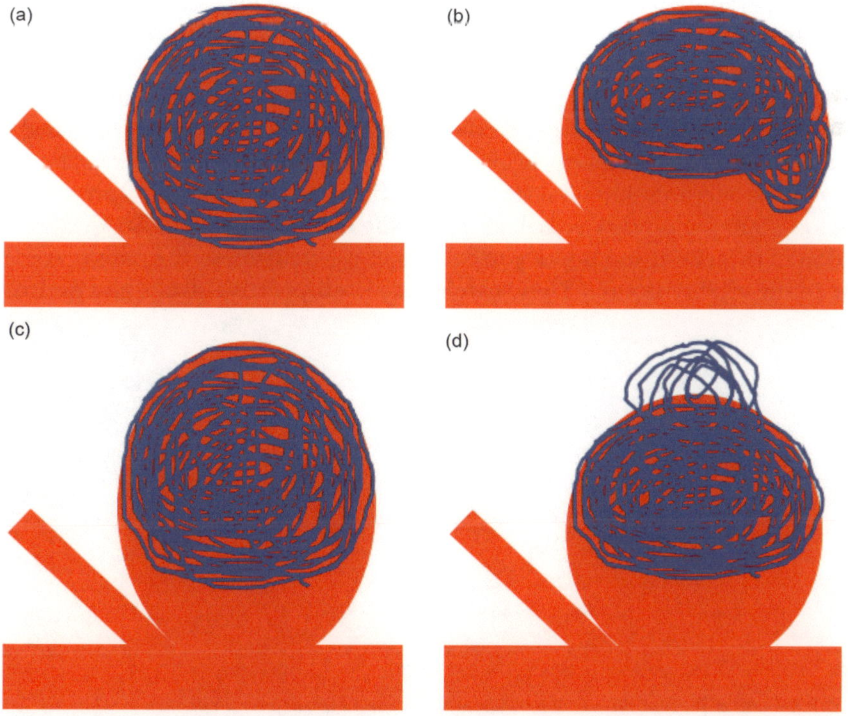

Figure 2.
(a)-(d): Schema of the mechanisms of the recurrence. (a): Complete obliteration of the aneurysm. (b): Coil compaction. (c): Aneurysm regrowth. (d): Fundal migration.

recurrent aneurysms after initial coil embolization with the stent, all patients had good outcomes (mRS 0-2), 16 patients had complete aneurysm occlusion, and one patient tended aneurysm regrowth [36]. Thus, the flow diverter, a novel treatment method, is currently a promising treatment option for recurrent cerebral aneurysms after initial coil embolization. Future case series and long-term follow-up studies are warranted.

In deciding the optimal treatment for patients with recurrent cerebral aneurysms after initial coil embolization, it is critical to consider the presence or absence of systemic complications comprehensively, the site of the aneurysms, and the mechanism of aneurysm recurrence in each case to determine the optimal treatment strategy.

6. Tips of direct surgery for recurrent aneurysms after endovascular coil embolization

When choosing open clipping of a recurrent cerebral aneurysm after initial coil embolization, it is critical to confirm by preoperative cerebral angiography that there is sufficient space between the neck and the coil mass to allow for clip application. (**Figure 3a** and **b**) Toyota et al. reported that a remnant neck height of the aneurysm more significant than 2 mm is a prerequisite for surgery if the coil mass within the aneurysm is not removed [37]. Also, Waldron et al. reported that open cerebral aneurysm clipping without removing the coil mass in the aneurysm is unsuitable when the coil width and compaction height ratio exceeds 2.5 and a wedge angle greater than 90 degrees [38]. Confirming these findings by preoperative cerebral angiography is essential.

Perioperative stroke complications have been reported to be higher in patients undergoing intraoperative coil mass extraction [23]. Coil extraction was performed in 3/111 patients (2.7%), all of whom suffered a postoperative stroke [39]. The effects of coil embolization of cerebral aneurysms on the vital structure of the aneurysm, mother vessel, branches, and cranial nerves have been attributed to inflammatory and degenerative change mechanisms. A coil mass within the aneurysm causes inflammation and degeneration, resulting in extrusion of the coil mass outside the aneurysm, invasion of the surrounding vital structure, inflammatory adhesions, protrusion of the coil loop into the mother vessel, and scarring of the vessel wall. Surgical coil mass extraction in this condition is likely to cause steno-occlusion of the parent artery and damage to the vital structure. These can lead to postoperative stroke and neurological

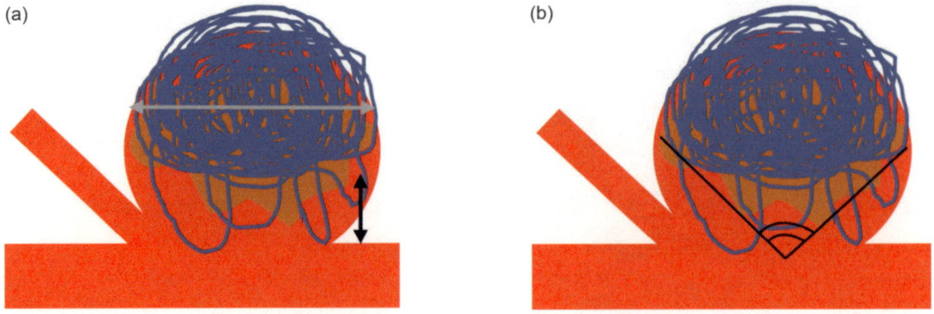

Figure 3.
(a) and (b): Schema of the morphological parameters of recurrent aneurysms after endovascular coil embolization. (a): The gray two-direction arrow indicates a coil width (C), and the black two-direction arrow indicates either a compaction height (H) or a remnant neck width (RNH). (b): The angle shown in the figure indicates a wedge angle. Aneurysms with RNH greater than 2 mm or a C/H ratio greater than 2.5 with a wedge angle greater than 90 degrees are unsuitable for direct clipping surgery without coil removal.

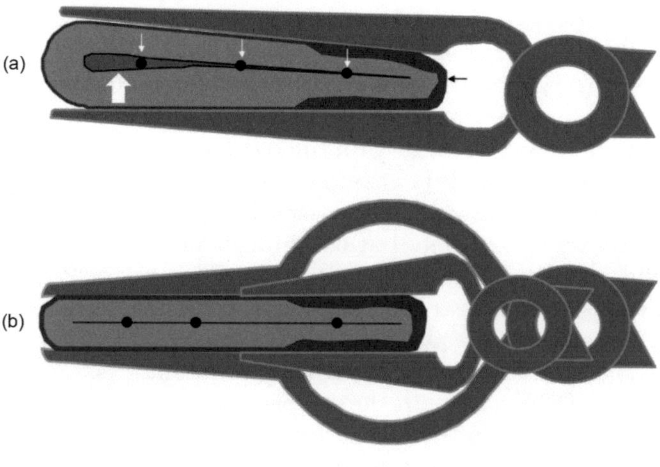

Figure 4.
a (upper) and b (lower): Schema of the neck clipping of the recurrence. (a): When a single aneurysm clip is applied to the aneurysm neck, atherosclerotic or inflammatory wall thickening (small black arrow) and coil loop inside (small white arrows) often prevent complete closure of the neck (thick white arrow). (b): The tandem clipping method, in which a fenestrated aneurysm clip is applied to the far side aneurysm neck, skipping the near side aneurysm neck, and an additional clip is used to close the near side aneurysm neck, is extremely useful in the above situation, as it provides complete closure of the neck.

sequelae. Therefore, in the case of open clipping of recurrent cerebral aneurysms after initial coil embolization, coil mass extraction should be avoided as much as possible to ensure a safe procedure with a low rate of surgical complications.

Even in cases where preoperative imaging has shown sufficient space for clip application in the recurrent cerebral aneurysm, intraoperative findings may indicate that the room is smaller than expected during surgery. This phenomenon may be due to thrombus formation caused by coil mass in the aneurysm or thickening of the aneurysm wall due to inflammatory changes. In addition, a coil loop in the neck of the aneurysm may prevent complete occlusion of the neck when a single clip is applied (**Figure 4a**). The tandem clipping method has been reported to help deal with incomplete occlusion of cerebral clips due to stiff neck aneurysm walls and coil loops (**Figure 4b**) [40]. In this technique, a fenestrated aneurysm clip is applied to the far side aneurysm neck, skipping the near side aneurysm neck, and an additional clip is used to close the near side aneurysm neck. This technique is beneficial in narrow aneurysm neck spaces, stiff aneurysm neck walls, and the presence of coil loops in the neck, as complete occlusion of the aneurysm neck can be achieved without coil mass extraction. On the other hand, for large or giant cerebral aneurysms that recur after initial coil embolization and are at high risk for open aneurysm clipping, mother vessel occlusion with intracranial or extracranial bypass may be helpful [38, 40]. By this surgical strategy, direct manipulation of the aneurysm is no longer necessary, and it can be a safe treatment for recurrent cerebral aneurysms after coil embolization of deep locations like the upper basilar artery system or when there is already a high mass effect on the vital structures.

7. Illustrative case presentations

Case 1: A 65-year-old woman presented with Hunt and Kosnik grade 1, Fisher group 3 subarachnoid hemorrhage. Her digital subtraction angiography (DSA) revealed a right internal carotid artery-posterior communicating (IC-Pcom) artery aneurysm. She underwent coil embolization. The aneurysm was completely obliterated. Her postoperative course was uneventful, and she was discharged home without a neurological deficit. Six months after initial treatment, follow-up DSA showed the remarkable recurrence of the aneurysm with coil compaction (**Figure 5a**). Thus, she underwent additional clipping surgery for the recurrent IC-Pcom aneurysm.

Intraoperative findings (Video 1 https://1drv.ms/f/s!AnNEb0cDd-ygmSdOw3kIA3vy_9kf?e=pgxew1): Coil mass inside the aneurysm dome were seen through not only the wall of the dome but also through the wall of the neck. First, we applied a straight-type titanium clip, but the tip slipped toward the Pcom, so we removed this clip. Then, we applied a fenestrated Elgiloy clip in partial occlusion of the far side aneurysm neck. Indocyanine-green video angiography (ICG-VA) showed patency of ICA, Pcom, and anterior choroidal artery and nonfilling of the aneurysm. We added a straight Elgiloy clip in parallel fashion to secure the complete obliteration of the aneurysm.

Postoperative CT showed no complication and complete obliteration of the aneurysm (**Figure 5b** and **c**). Her postoperative course was uneventful, and she was discharged home without a neurological deficit.

Case 2: A 63-year-old woman presented with Hunt and Kosnik grade 2, Fisher group 3 subarachnoid hemorrhage. Her DSA revealed a right IC-Pcom artery aneurysm. She underwent coil embolization. The aneurysm was completely obliterated. Her postoperative course was uneventful, and she was discharged home without a neurological deficit. Forty-one months after initial treatment, follow-up DSA showed the remarkable recurrence of the aneurysm with fundal migration (**Figure 6a**). Thus, she underwent additional clipping surgery for the recurrent IC-Pcom aneurysm.

Intraoperative findings (**Video 2** https://1drv.ms/f/s!AnNEb0cDd-ygmSdOw3kIA3vy_9kf?e=FQyE2p): Coil mass inside the aneurysm dome were seen through the dome's wall. And fundal migrated coil loops compressed the right oculomotor nerve. We applied a straight-type titanium clip to the neck of the aneurysm and supposed this to be complete obliteration. We incised the dome with microscissors to release the oculomotor nerve from compression by the coil loops. Major bleeding was seen from the incised aneurysm dome. To stop bleeding, we applied a temporary clip to the proximal ICA. The bleeding was controlled completely. Then we applied an additional fenestrated clip and removed the temporary clip.

Postoperative CT showed a thin epidural hematoma and complete aneurysm obliteration (**Figure 6b** and **c**). Her postoperative course was uneventful, and she was discharged home without a neurological deficit.

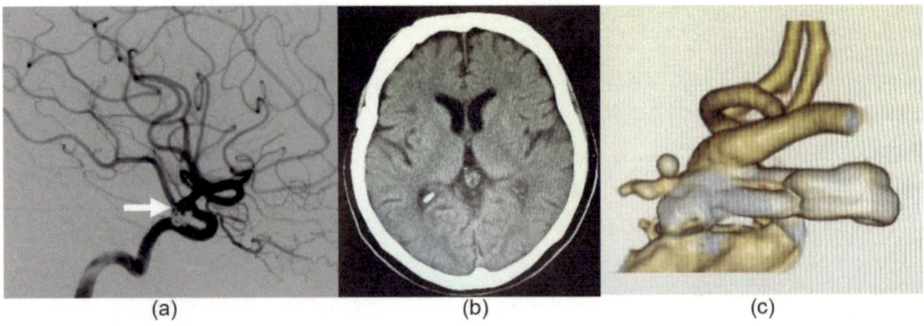

Figure 5.
a-c: The imaging studies of illustrative case 1. (a): Follow-up DSA (lateral view of right ICGA) 6 months after initial coil embolization showed remarkable recurrence of the treated IC-Pcom aneurysm (white arrow). (b) and (c): Postoperative plain CT and CT angiography showed no complication and complete obliteration of the aneurysm.

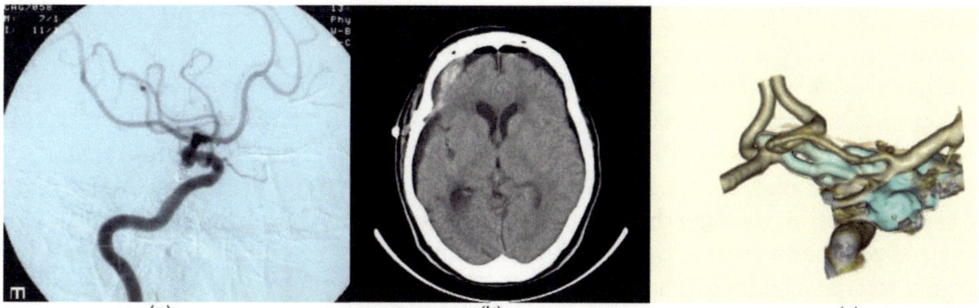

(a) (b) (c)

Figure 6.
a-c the imaging studies of illustrative case 2. (a) Follow-up DSA (lateral view of right ICGA) 41 months after initial coil embolization showed remarkable recurrence of the treated IC-Pcom aneurysm (white arrow). (b) and (c) postoperative plain CT and CT angiography showed thin epidural hematoma and complete aneurysm obliteration.

Case 3: A 43-year-old man presented with Hunt and Kosnik grade 3, Fisher group 3 subarachnoid hemorrhage. His DSA revealed a left IC-Pcom artery aneurysm. He underwent coil embolization. The aneurysm was completely obliterated. His postoperative course was uneventful, and he was discharged home without a neurological deficit. Eighteen months after initial treatment, follow-up DSA showed the remarkable recurrence of the aneurysm with regrowth, and he underwent additional stent-assisted coil embolization for the aneurysm. However, 30 months after the second treatment, follow-up MRI and DSA revealed the recurrence as a partially thrombosed

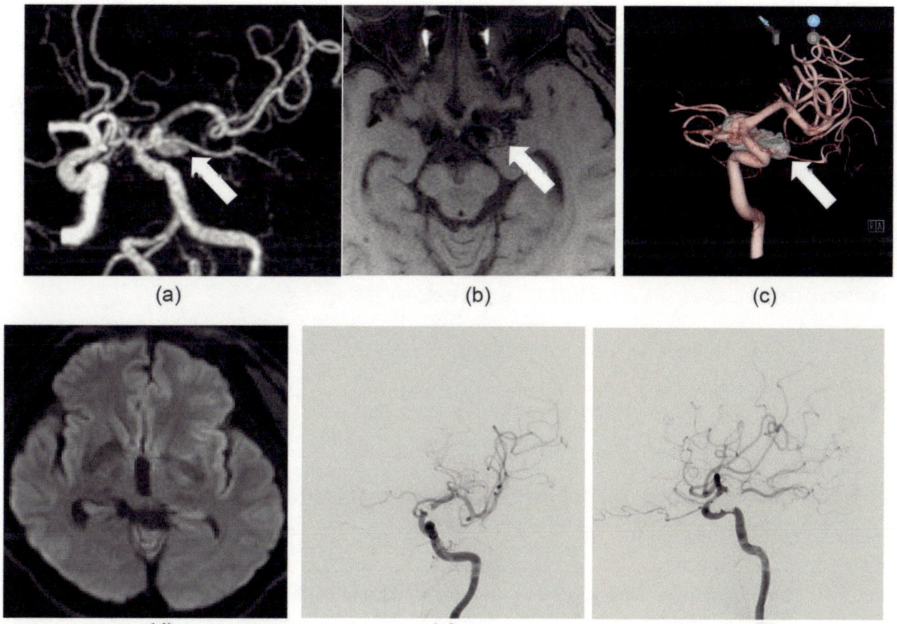

(a) (b) (c)

(d) (e) (f)

Figure 7.
a-f: The preoperative (a-c) and postoperative (d-f) imaging studies of illustrative case 3. (a) Silent MRA 30 months after the second treatment. (b) T1-weighted MRI. (c) 3D rotational angiography. The imaging studies showed recurrent partially thrombosed giant left IC-Pcom aneurysm (white arrow). (d) Postoperative diffusion-weighted MRI. (e) and (f): Postoperative DSA anterior-posterior and lateral view. The imaging studies showed no ischemic complication and complete aneurysm obliteration with preservation of normal arteries.

giant aneurysm (**Figure 7a–c**). Thus, he underwent additional clipping surgery for the recurrent IC-Pcom aneurysm.

Intraoperative findings (Video 3 https://1drv.ms/v/s!AnNEb0cDd-ygmSsspZ6yOvo4Mle1?e=hlee0e): The stent was inserted in the left proximal intracranial ICA, but proximal control at this site was confirmed feasible. Left Pcom origin was observed at the proximal neck of the aneurysm. Coil mass inside the aneurysm dome and stent strut were seen through the wall of the dome and ICA. The left anterior choroidal artery and perforators from Pcom firmly adhered to the dome of the aneurysm. The adhesion was detached with sharp dissection. While performing temporary occlusion in the proximal intracranial ICA, first, we applied a fenestrated titanium clip in partial occlusion of the far side aneurysm neck. ICG-VA revealed the residual flow into the aneurysm through the near side of the neck of the aneurysm. We added a straight titanium clip in a parallel fashion to secure the complete obliteration of the aneurysm. ICG-VA showed complete obliteration of the aneurysm and preservation of the parent artery and branches.

Postoperative imaging studies showed complete aneurysm obliteration without complication (**Figure 7d–f**). His postoperative course was uneventful, and he was discharged home without a neurological deficit.

8. Conclusions

The role of craniotomy in treating recurrent cerebral aneurysms after initial coil embolization has been discussed in detail. The optimal treatment strategy for this lesion should be decided based on the location of the aneurysm, the mechanism of recurrence, the presence or absence of systemic complications, and the performance status of the individual patient. In the case of recurrence by aneurysmal regrowth mechanisms, the choice of direct surgery leads to a low recurrence rate. In direct surgery, clipping without coil mass extraction is safer. The tandem clipping method is a beneficial technique that can achieve complete occlusion of these aneurysms.

Conflict of interest

The author declares no conflict of interest.

Author details

Tsuyoshi Izumo
Department of Neurosurgery, Nagasaki University Graduate School of Biomedical Sciences, Nagasaki, Japan

*Address all correspondence to: go-izumo@hotmail.co.jp

References

[1] Cohen-Gadol AA, Spencer DD, Harvey W. Cushing and cerebrovascular surgery: Part I, aneurysms. Journal of Neurosurgery. 2004;**101**(3):547-552

[2] Mount LA. Results of treatment of intracranial aneurysms using the Selverstone clamp. Journal of Neurosurgery. 1959;**16**:611-618

[3] Horiuchi T, Ito K, Hongo K, Shibuya M. Mechanical evaluation of long titanium alloy clip: Comparison of cobalt alloy clip. Neurologia Medico-Chirurgica (Tokyo). 2013;**54**(3):176-179

[4] Horiuchi T, Rahmah NN, Yanagawa T, Hongo K. Revisit of aneurysm clip closing forces: Comparison of titanium versus cobalt alloy clip. Neurosurgical Review. 2013;**36**(1):133-137 discussion 7-8

[5] Ebina K, Iwabuchi T, Suzuki S. Histological change in permanently clipped or ligated cerebral arterial wall. Part I. an experimental study in dogs. Acta Neurochirurgica. 1982;**65**(3-4):253-276

[6] Izumo T, Morofuji Y, Hayashi K, Ryu N, Matsuo T. Surgical treatment of ruptured anterior circulation aneurysms: Comparative analysis of modified mini-Pterional and standard Pterional craniotomies. Neurology India. 2019;**67**(5):1248-1253

[7] Hopf NJ, Stadie A, Reisch R. Surgical management of bilateral middle cerebral artery aneurysms via a unilateral supraorbital key-hole craniotomy. Minimally Invasive Neurosurgery: MIN. 2009;**52**(3):126-131

[8] Hughes-Hallett A, Mayer EK, Pratt PJ, Vale JA, Darzi AW. Quantitative analysis of technological innovation in minimally invasive surgery. The British Journal of Surgery. 2015;**102**(2):e151-e157

[9] Solomon RA, Fukushima T. New aneurysm clip appliers for "key-hole" neurosurgery. Neurosurgery. 1991;**28**(3):474-476

[10] Siddique K, Alvernia J, Fraser K, Lanzino G. Treatment of aneurysms with wires and electricity: A historical overview. Journal of Neurosurgery. 2003;**99**(6):1102-1107

[11] Benati A, Maschio A, Perini S, Beltramello A. Treatment of posttraumatic carotid-cavernous fistula using a detachable balloon catheter. Journal of Neurosurgery. 1980;**53**(6):784-786

[12] Debrun G, Lacour P, Caron JP, Hurth M, Comoy J, Keravel Y. Detachable balloon and calibrated-leak balloon techniques in the treatment of cerebral vascular lesions. Journal of Neurosurgery. 1978;**49**(5):635-649

[13] Romodanov SA, Sheglov VI. Preoperative occlusion by detachable balloon catheter of the arteries feeding meningiomas of supratentorial location. Klinicheskaia Khirurgiia. 1962;**1979**(7):41-44

[14] Taki W, Handa H, Yonekawa Y, Yamagata S, Miyake H, Matsuda I, et al. Detachable balloon catheter systems for embolization of cerebrovascular lesions. Neurologia Medico-Chirurgica (Tokyo). 1981;**21**(7):709-719

[15] Guglielmi G, Viñuela F, Sepetka I, Macellari V. Electrothrombosis of saccular aneurysms via endovascular approach. Part 1: Electrochemical basis, technique, and experimental results. Journal of Neurosurgery. 1991;**75**(1):1-7

[16] Molyneux A, Kerr R, Stratton I, Sandercock P, Clarke M, Shrimpton J, et al. International subarachnoid aneurysm trial (ISAT) of neurosurgical clipping versus endovascular coiling in 2143 patients with ruptured intracranial aneurysms: A randomized trial. Journal of Stroke and Cerebrovascular Diseases. 2002;**11**(6):304-314

[17] Spetzler RF, McDougall CG, Zabramski JM, Albuquerque FC, Hills NK, Russin JJ, et al. The Barrow ruptured aneurysm trial: 6-year results. Journal of Neurosurgery. 2015;**123**(3):609-617

[18] Zaidi HA, Montoure A, Elhadi A, Nakaji P, McDougall CG, Albuquerque FC, et al. Long-term functional outcomes and predictors of shunt-dependent hydrocephalus after treatment of ruptured intracranial aneurysms in the BRAT trial: Revisiting the clip vs coil debate. Neurosurgery. 2015;**76**(5):608-615

[19] Huang H, Limb R, Lai LT. Is it time to rethink microsurgical training for the treatment of intracranial aneurysms in Australia? Journal of Clinical Neuroscience. 2023;**108**:95-101

[20] Beydoun HA, Beydoun M, Zonderman A, Eid SM. Perioperative ischemic stroke in Unruptured intracranial aneurysm surgical or endovascular therapy. Cureus. 2020;**12**(4):e7645

[21] Stapleton CJ, Walcott BP, Butler WE, Ogilvy CS. Neurological outcomes following intraprocedural rerupture during coil embolization of ruptured intracranial aneurysms. Journal of Neurosurgery. 2015;**122**(1):128-135

[22] Arnaout OM, El Ahmadieh TY, Zammar SG, El Tecle NE, Hamade YJ, Aoun RJ, et al. Microsurgical treatment of previously coiled intracranial aneurysms: Systematic review of the literature. World Neurosurgery. 2015;**84**(2):246-253

[23] Petr O, Brinjikji W, Thomé C, Lanzino G. Safety and efficacy of microsurgical treatment of previously coiled aneurysms: A systematic review and meta-analysis. Acta Neurochirurgica. 2015;**157**(10):1623-1632

[24] Zhang G, Wu Y, Wei Y, Xue G, Chen R, Lv N, et al. Stent-assisted coiling vs. coiling alone of ruptured tiny intracranial aneurysms: A contemporary cohort study in a high-volume center. Frontiers in Neurology. 2022;**13**:1076026

[25] Fuga M, Tanaka T, Irie K, Kajiwara I, Tachi R, Teshigawara A, et al. Risk factors for recanalization of dense coil packing for unruptured cerebral aneurysms in endovascular coil embolization: Analysis of a single center's experience. Journal of Clinical Neuroscience. 2022;**98**:175-181

[26] Caratinvestigators. Rates of delayed rebleeding from intracranial aneurysms are low after surgical and endovascular treatment. Stroke. 2006;**37**:1437-1442

[27] Daou MR, El Ahmadieh TY, El Tecle NE, Bohnen AM, Bendok BR. Unruptured intracranial aneurysms: Risk factors and their interactions. Neurosurgery. 2013;**73**:N14-N15

[28] Byrne JV, Sohn MJ, Molyneux AJ, Chir B. Five-year experience in using coil embolization for ruptured intracranial aneurysms: Outcomes and incidence of late rebleeding. Journal of Neurosurgery. 1999;**90**(4):656-663

[29] Dorfer C, Gruber A, Standhardt H, Bavinzski G, Knosp E. Management of residual and recurrent aneurysms after initial endovascular treatment. Neurosurgery. 2012;**70**(3):537-553 discussion 53-4

[30] Campi A, Ramzi N, Molyneux AJ, Summers PE, Kerr RS, Sneade M, et al. Retreatment of ruptured cerebral aneurysms in patients randomized by coiling or clipping in the international subarachnoid aneurysm trial (ISAT). Stroke. 2007;**38**(5):1538-1544

[31] Ries T, Siemonsen S, Thomalla G, Grzyska U, Zeumer H, Fiehler J. Long-term follow-up of cerebral aneurysms after endovascular therapy prediction and outcome of retreatment. AJNR. American Journal of Neuroradiology. 2007;**28**(9):1755-1761

[32] Lee J, Lim JW, Cho YD. Follow-up outcomes after Re-embolization for recanalized aneurysms after initial coiling: Further recurrence rates and related risk factors. World Neurosurgery. 2018;**114**:e508-ee17

[33] Kang HS, Han MH, Kwon BJ, Kwon OK, Kim SH. Repeat endovascular treatment in post-embolization recurrent intracranial aneurysms. Neurosurgery. 2006;**58**(1):60-70 discussion 60-70

[34] Kang HS, Kwon BJ, Kim JE, Han MH. Preinterventional clopidogrel response variability for coil embolization of intracranial aneurysms: Clinical implications. AJNR. American Journal of Neuroradiology. 2010;**31**(7):1206-1210

[35] Li W, Zhu W, Sun X, Liu J, Wang Y, Wang K, et al. Retreatment with flow diverters and coiling for recurrent aneurysms after initial endovascular treatment: A propensity score-matched comparative analysis. Frontiers in Neurology. 2021;**12**:625652

[36] Park KY, Yeon JY, Kim BM, Jeon P, Kim JH, Jang CK, et al. Efficacy and safety of flow-diverter therapy for recurrent aneurysms after stent-assisted coiling. AJNR. American Journal of Neuroradiology. 2020;**41**(4):663-668

[37] Toyota S, Taki T, Wakayama A, Yoshimine T. Retreatment of recurrent internal carotid-posterior communicating artery aneurysm after coil embolization. Neurologia Medico-Chirurgica (Tokyo). 2015;**55**(11):838-847

[38] Waldron JS, Halbach VV, Lawton MT. Microsurgical management of incompletely coiled and recurrent aneurysms: Trends, techniques, and observations on coil extrusion. Neurosurgery. 2009;**64**(5 Suppl 2):301-315 discussion 15-7

[39] Daou B, Chalouhi N, Starke RM, Barros G, Ya'qoub L, Do J, et al. Clipping of previously coiled cerebral aneurysms: Efficacy, safety, and predictors in a cohort of 111 patients. Journal of Neurosurgery. 2016;**125**(6):1337-1343

[40] Izumo T, Matsuo T, Morofuji Y, Hiu T, Horie N, Hayashi K, et al. Microsurgical clipping for recurrent aneurysms after initial endovascular coil embolization. World Neurosurgery. 2015;**83**(2):211-218